Ethical Hospital Branding & Marketing

notionpress
.com

INDIA • SINGAPORE • MALAYSIA

Ethical Hospital Branding & Marketing

15 PROVEN STRATEGIES TO BUILD YOUR BRAND BOTH ONLINE & OFFLINE

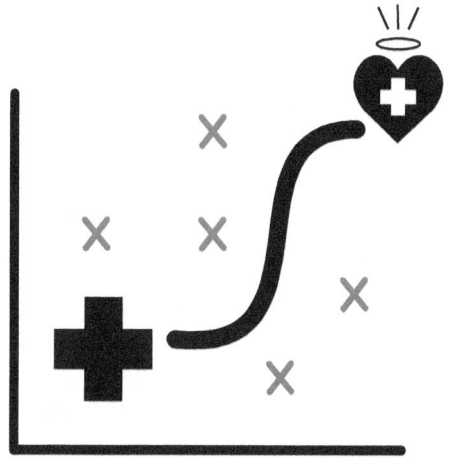

BUILD YOUR BRAND. BUILD YOUR LEGACY
MOHAMMED ILIAS

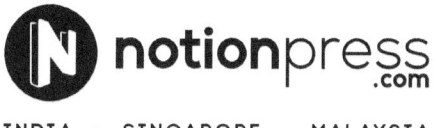

INDIA • SINGAPORE • MALAYSIA

Notion Press

No.8, 3rd Cross Street,
CIT Colony, Mylapore,
Chennai, Tamil Nadu – 600004

First Published by Notion Press 2021
Copyright © Mohammed Ilias 2021
All Rights Reserved.

ISBN 978-1-63745-519-7

This book has been published with all efforts taken to make the material error-free after the consent of the author. However, the author and the publisher do not assume and hereby disclaim any liability to any party for any loss, damage, or disruption caused by errors or omissions, whether such errors or omissions result from negligence, accident, or any other cause.

While every effort has been made to avoid any mistake or omission, this publication is being sold on the condition and understanding that neither the author nor the publishers or printers would be liable in any manner to any person by reason of any mistake or omission in this publication or for any action taken or omitted to be taken or advice rendered or accepted on the basis of this work. For any defect in printing or binding the publishers will be liable only to replace the defective copy by another copy of this work then available.

*To my Mom, Dad, Wife & Kids
and Also to Raja (My Business Partner)*

*Special Thanks to Keerthana for valuable support
in content and Jayaganesh, Kamlesh & William
for the book designing - wrapper, illustrations, and
infographics.*

*Thanks to the valuable support provided by my clients
and friends from medical fraternity in helping me
understand the hospital business dynamics without
whose help this book wouldn't be possible.*

CONTENTS

pg

STRATEGY 1
**"Don't battle with their Minds,
Win their hearts with a Cause"**
CAUSE BASED MARKETING — 01

STRATEGY 2
**"When your presence is strongly felt,
your purpose is fairly met"**
PERSONAL BRANDING — 19

STRATEGY 3
**"A man without a face is
same as a brand without logo"**
LOGO DESIGN & POSITIONING — 41

STRATEGY 4
"Your Network is Your Net worth"
WORD-OF-MOUTH — 55

STRATEGY 5
**"The more real it is,
the more reliable it gets!"**
PATIENT EXPERIENCE — 67

CONTENTS

pg

STRATEGY 6
"The Digital Future is NOW. Play it as it evolves!"
DIGITAL MARKETING — 83

STRATEGY 7
"Success creates more success when you make success reach"
CASE STUDY — 133

STRATEGY 8
"Their journey, defines your brand story"
PATIENT JOURNEY MAPPING — 143

STRATEGY 9
"Look beyond borders, the WORLD needs you!"
INTERNATIONAL PATIENTS — 153

STRATEGY 10
"Redefine your Targets, Redefine your Markets"
REBRANDING — 165

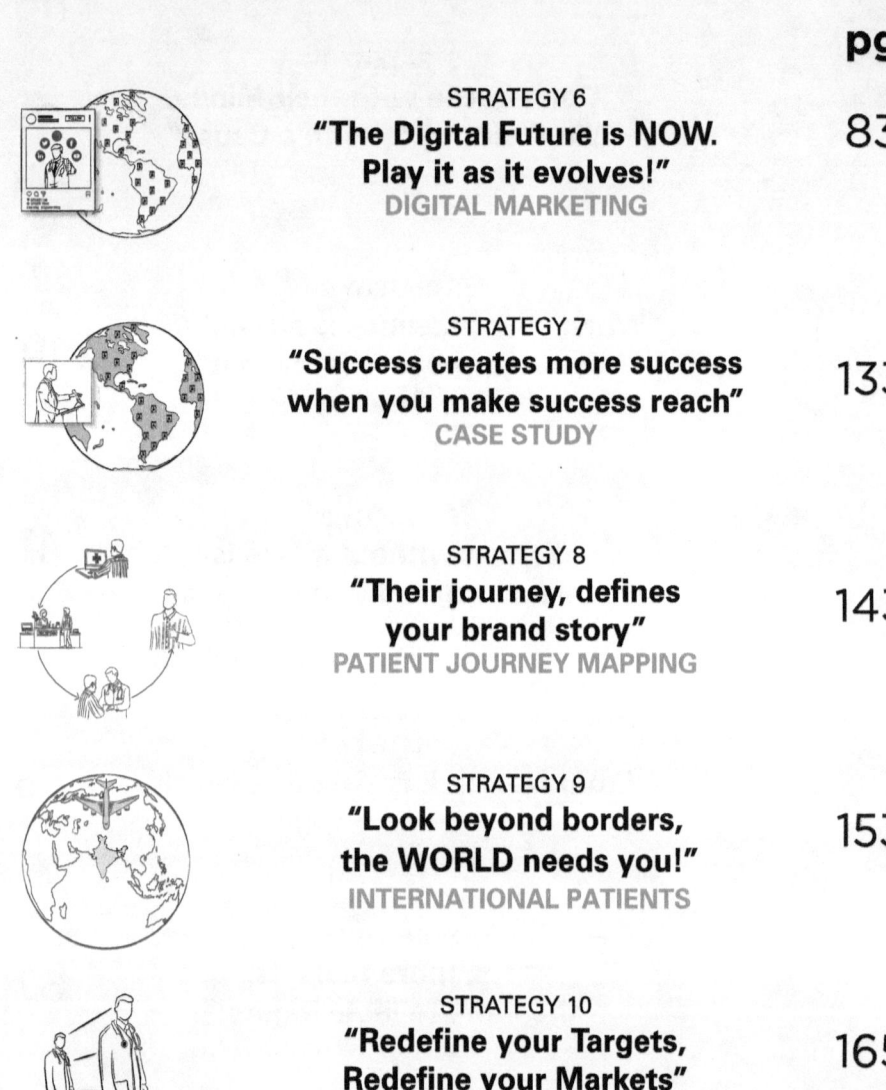

CONTENTS

		pg
	STRATEGY 11 **"By making others win, you win Big"** COLLABORATION	**175**
	STRATEGY 12 **"Local Hero is the one who is close to heart"** LOCAL MARKETING	**181**
	STRATEGY 13 **"Your Niche is your way to your glory and success"** Specialty SPECIFIC	**193**
	STRATEGY 14 **"Create your own tribe and lead them"** BUILD YOUR AUDIENCE	**203**
	STRATEGY 15 **"Know yourself before others know you"** REPUTATION MANAGEMENT	**213**

Ethical Hospital Branding & Marketing

15 PROVEN STRATEGIES TO BUILD YOUR BRAND BOTH ONLINE & OFFLINE

INTRODUCTION

Is Marketing a bad word in healthcare? I dont think so.

Marketing has a Noble Responsibility!

Governments spend billions of dollars on marketing health awareness to safeguard people against deadly diseases. It's all about the rightful use of marketing that matters. why do they depend on marketing? Because they know only through the rightful use of marketing, these life-saving messages can reach the masses in no time and save them. If one can dig deeper and understand, it is not marketing, which is bad but human greed. The real nature of marketing is pure - it has all the essentials in making good, reach people faster. Then, where have we gone wrong - its the approach that matters.

Hospitals using retail formats in marketing communication is not a welcome move; in fact, it degrades their brand when people start observing discounts, camps & master health checkups as baits, they lose faith in the hospital.

Hospital Marketing is not to create hype but to genuinely help people. No one lives in this world without needing healthcare, but what has to be understood is how you build trust with your marketing communication so that they come to you when they are in need. Marketing in its own nature need is not pushy.

This book aims to throw light on the true nature of hospital marketing, which is not revealed to hospital owners/ administrators/ marketers before in this format, the traces of which can be found in many places, but one book that covers it all is here before you.

Strategies discussed here are very powerful when implemented, volumes can be written explaining each one in detail but that wont help - this book gives all these strategies for you in a nutshell with an activity plan to use. You can expand the use of these strategies, don't just confine yourself to its limited applications mentioned in this book. And I would be happy to learn from you on the productive use of these strategies implemented in your style - please do share your learnings and results.

I have laid out 15 Ethical Strategies to brand and market your hospital. All these well laid out strategies will guide you on how to make your brand powerful, helpful, trusted, and loved by people. You will also learn how to build your brand audience and lead them by helping them experience "Moments of Truth" who will become your active word-of-mouth brand advocates, they will believe you and promote you.

Use these strategies to build a brand that you will be proud of, your generation and your next generation, generations after that will be proud of. A brand that will be considered a savior / a messiah by people who are just waiting for you. Take charge and help them.

Build your Brand!
Build your Legacy!!

STRATEGY 1

"DON'T BATTLE WITH THEIR MINDS, WIN THEIR HEARTS WITH A CAUSE"

CAUSE BASED MARKETING

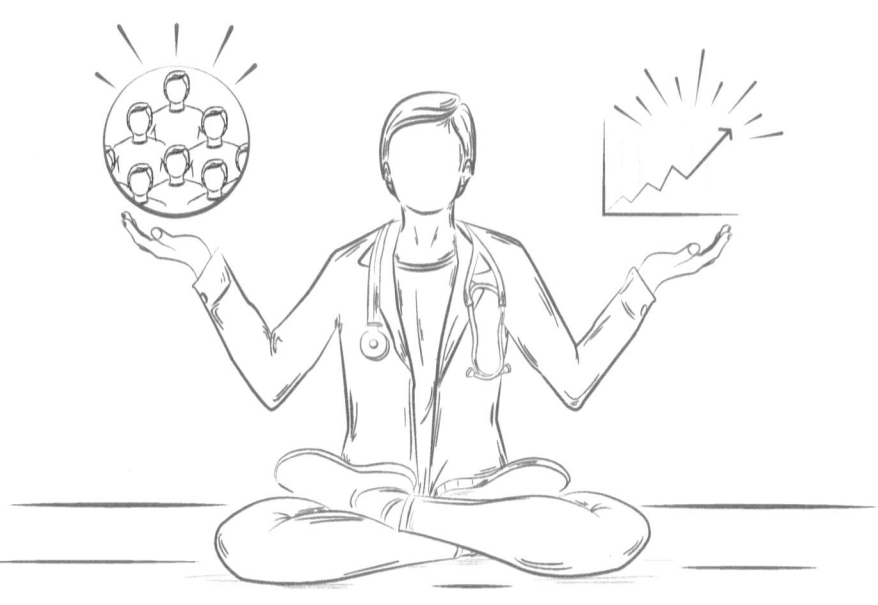

Begin with a cause

The more the market develops, the more mature it becomes with a lot of information aiming at different benefits. If you think you are a healthcare brand that deserves attention, importance, and respect then so, are other healthcare brands thinking about themselves. How do you think you will cut through the crowd or get where you want to get to. The way forward is by extending compassion beyond your profession.

We, as a society, are in deep need of solution givers and saviors who can promote healthy living in noble ways. Such acts should start from within, you have a wand in your hands to pass on the effect of healing to the whole world through your profession. Don't restrict the difference it can make to this world.

It is your responsibility to ensure that people around you are hale and healthy irrespective of them being your patients or not. So go ahead, put that foot forward as a responsible healthcare brand and make the actual difference you are meant to be making. Cause based approach will take any healthcare brand closer to what it is set out to be in a short while than the brand predicted for itself, as the noble cause of spreading awareness, precaution giving, treating and healing people will become more accessible through your cause campaigns.

Touch people, remember the world doesn't fall for moving images but images that move. If you really care for people around you then you need to tell them that you do. They'll love your healthcare brand more than ever.

Take the best road to craft a brand image for yourself. There are different approaches to market a healthcare brand, each one significant on their own promise to give out a result that positively impacts the motive of the healthcare brand. But choosing that one approach that is all set to give you the right benefits like activating the welfare motive behind your healthcare brand, getting more close to your target audience, standing up tall for causes and concentrating on big problems your healthcare brand is set to solve will all be met at once when you choose Cause Based Marketing.

Understanding the very concept of Cause Based Marketing

Cause based marketing is the process of gracefully blending a cause to your business goals. Marketing a cause along with your organizational capabilities and increasing your brand awareness among people by reaching them for a purpose. Choose Cause Based Marketing to increase the intimacy between your brand loyalists and your brand. While you promote a cause you are making your brand more accessible to people who want to get closer to you. Standing up for a cause as a brand contributes to your healthcare brand image.

Cause Based Marketing has its own way of leveraging your healthcare brand's presence and impression in the market by highlighting the good nature of your healthcare brand. Also, the primary motto of any healthcare brand is to put its patients first which will be proven with added trust factors from the patient's side when a healthcare brand adopts a Cause Based Marketing approach.

10 Commandments of Cause Based Marketing

1. The noble profession needs noble ways of promotion

Cause Based marketing is the most compassionate way to promote compassion in your healthcare business. Cause Based Marketing campaigns can leverage the healthcare brand value and increase its awareness among potential patients. Cause Based Marketing uses the goodness to create more goodness through working on it. Noble way of marketing your healthcare brand is required to cut through the chaos and reach your target audience.

2. Select a cause dear to you, not your competitor

A Cause Based Marketing campaign is primarily defined by the cause itself. The cause should align with your strategy and brand goal, be it long term or short term and not just a mere imitation of what your competing brand is following. So choose your cause wisely. Every healthcare brand is unique in its own way, embrace the uniqueness. Choose a cause that matters the most to your healthcare brand.

3. Promote your brand in the run of promoting your cause, NOT vice-versa

Promoting the cause and creating a healthier society through your campaign should be your main goal. Your cause is your hero so that it naturally brings your brand to the limelight. Don't let your brand and its capabilities overwhelm your Cause Based Marketing campaign. Promote a cause with utmost honesty and reach the maximum through your honest motive. So, the good deeds add on to your healthcare brand's social merit and desirability.

4 Invest more than just money

There is a lot that goes into your Cause Based Marketing campaign than just the piece of marketing budget allocated. Make your marketing budget according to how you have segmented your target audience pertaining to the cause. In Cause Based Marketing one-size-fits-all solution will generally not work. You being the sole carrier of the message will not multiply the reach of the cause as much as you want it to. So, bring on a battalion of cause promoters with an appropriate proportion of medical and non-medical staff, make necessary arrangements based on the nature of the campaign consult experts to conceptualize and strategize.

5 A share in hearts is greater than a mere share in the market

The biggest significance of a Cause Based Marketing campaign is that it can give a great edge in terms of preference among your potential patient base as they already know your brand for the goodness it creates and spreads. Your community knows you for your compassion. People need that feeling of their own while handing over the responsibility of their well being to your healthcare brand, this yarn of familiarity can be spun by Cause Based Marketing approach only..

6 Select a cause that is dear to your specialty

Your choice of cause can be a chance to play your strengths to your advantage. A cause that directly relates to your specialty discipline will make your Cause Based Marketing campaign stronger and will result in making your services reach the right people.

7. Make alliances that make you matter

Join hands with the biggies of the cause you have chosen. If you see a campaign by worldwide healthcare organizations like UNESCO, join hands with them and add to the voice they are trying to create in your surroundings, by doing so you earn more merit and a share of their credibility. Join hands with NGOs who are also fighting on a similar cause - through the right collaboration you can get the right visibility. The right collaboration will also give you the right strength to move forward and serve those in need.

8. Help in Emergencies, Epidemics, and Controversies

Unfortunate outbreak of new diseases that people are unaware of and not used to managing is a crisis that only your fraternity could manage. The healthcare industry can send awareness messages or cautions at the time of such outbreaks to de-stress people. Let your Cause Based messages clear the air and send authentic bulletins and instructions for people to follow. Giving clear cut prevention and cure instructions will sow your brand image deeply in people's minds. They will remember you for your timely help. Remember that your service gets a greater value when it can touch lives at the right time.

9. Sincerity shows and so does insincerity

Don't consider Caused Based Marketing is about using the cause as bait to promote your practice/hospital - in such way Cause Based Marketing does not work. People can see skin deep today and understand what the truth is. This approach is sincerely doing good i.e. genuinely marrying a cause into your practice.

Use your PR wisely, instruct them on the tone, nature and the extent of brand promotion that should be included while they cover your Cause Based Marketing event. The genuineness of your healthcare brand should be the best part of Cause Based Marketing.

10 Create a system so that the good continues

Create a system that brings alive the action you advocated for, push the cause forward even after your campaign is over so that the real compassion of your healthcare brand is given a chance to change the world. Make your awareness campaigns reach as many as possible who are interested in making the world a better place to live. Let Cause Based Marketing make a real change in your immediate surroundings, then you will see how effective your healthcare brand can get. And create a system so that the good continues long after the cause campaign was started and becomes more mature with time.

Cause Based Marketing is the approach to make any healthcare brand connect to people strongly at a personal level. Touch people's hearts for once, they will remember you and get reminded of you a million times and will also tell others. That is the way a healthcare brand has to really progress, it is not just a mere growth in terms of numbers as healthcare itself is a very very personal and noble profession sometimes looked as mere messiah, savior or an ultimate power in the universe. So take the responsibility on your shoulder and play your part. Let your healthcare brand make an exact difference on earth that it is born to make, for the world will thank you forever.

1
CAUSE BASED MARKETING
ACTION PLAN

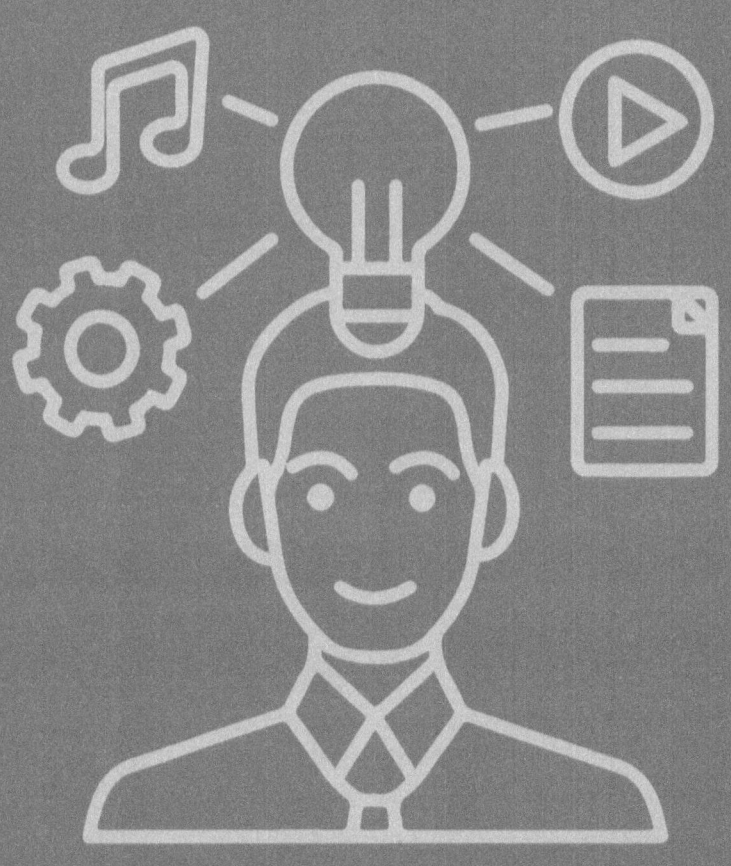

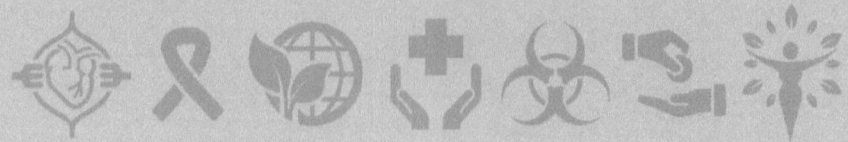

7 TYPES OF CAUSE BASED CAMPAIGNS

PICK THE ONE THAT SUITS YOU BETTER

01 SPECIALTY CAUSE CAMPAIGN
Cause that is related to your area of specialization

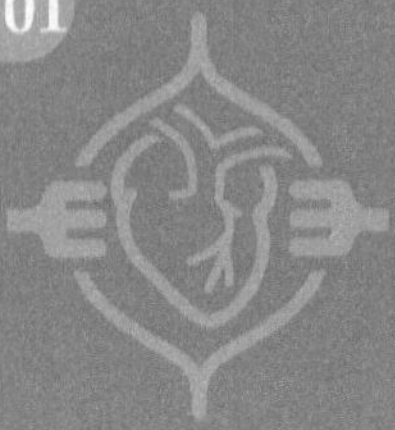

Eg: Heart Campaign for Heart Day with Cardiology as your area of specialization.

02 SOCIAL CAUSE CAMPAIGN
Causes that challenge the social taboos and myths in society

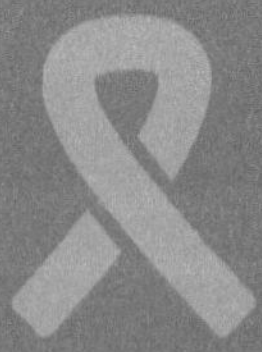

Eg: Infertility awareness campaign that help people break out of unscientific beliefs.

03 ENVIRONMENTAL CAUSE CAMPAIGN
Causes that relate to health issues caused due to environmental conditions.

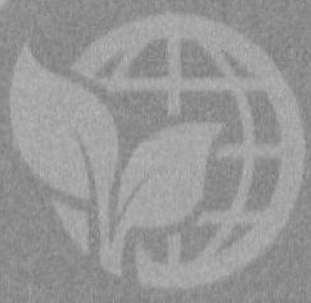

Eg: Awareness campaigns against environmental pollution.

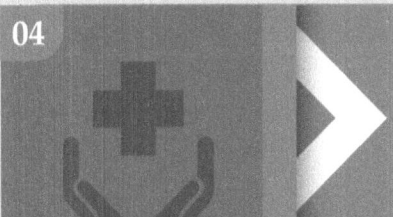 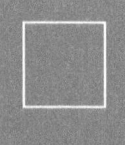

PUBLIC HEALTH CAUSE CAMPAIGN

Causes that relate to general public health and well being

Eg: Stop Smoking Campaign.

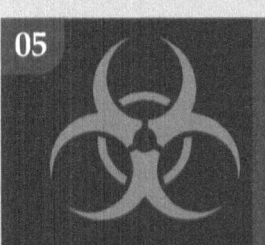  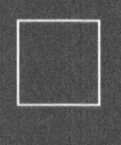

EPIDEMIC CAUSE CAMPAIGN

Causes that relate to saving people from epidemics and crisis communication.

Eg: Corona Virus (Covid-19) prevention programs

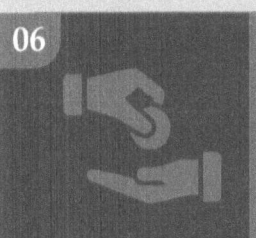 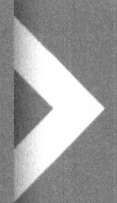 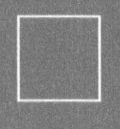

FUND RAISING CAUSE CAMPAIGN

Causes that related to raising funds for needy patients.

Eg: Public appeal with patient case scenario & procedure cost estimate

 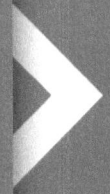 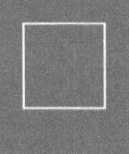

WOMEN WELLNESS CAUSE CAMPAIGN

Causes that are specific & related to wellness of women.

Eg: Cervical Cancer & Breast Cancer awareness programs

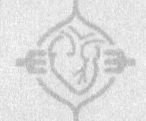 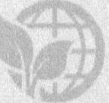 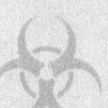 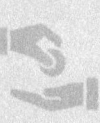 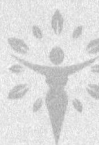

HEALTHCARE AWARENESS DAY
CALENDAR

JAN	**01-31** National Birth Defects Prevention Month	**18-24** Pap Smear Week

FEB	**04** World Cancer Day	**08** International Epilepsy Day	**07-14** National Healthy Marriage Week	**15** International Childhood Cancer Day

MAR	**01-31** Colorectal Cancer Awareness Month	**03** World Hearing Day	**04** World obesity day	**11** World Kidney Day
	20 World Oral Health Day	**21** World Down Syndrome Day	**24** World Tuberculosis (TB) Day	

APR	**02** World Autism Awareness Day	**07** World Health Day	**24-30** World Immunization Week

MAY	**04** World Asthma Day	**08** World Thalassemia Day	**17** World Hypertension Day	**30** World MS Day
				31 World No Tobacco Day

JUN	**14** World Blood Donor Day	**19** World Sickle Cell Day	**21** International Yoga Day

HEALTHCARE AWARENESS DAY
CALENDAR

JUL
- **01** Happy Doctors Day
- **14** India Population Control Contraception Promotion Day
- **28** World Hepatitis Day

AUG
- **01-07** World Breastfeeding Week
- **06-07** Infertility Day

SEP
- **04** World Sexual Health Day
- **14** World First Aid Day
- **21** World Alzheimer's Day
- **29** World Heart Day

OCT
- **01-31** Breast Cancer Awareness Month
- **01** International Day of Older Persons
- **10** World Mental Health Day
- **12** World Arthritis Day
- **12-18** International Infection Prevention Week
- **15** Global Handwashing Day
- **20** World Osteoporosis Day
- **24** World Polio Day

NOV
- **01-29** Lung Cancer Awareness Month
- **14** World Diabetes Day
- **17** World Prematurity Day
- **21** World COPD Day
- **18-24** World Antibiotic Awareness Week
- **20** World Children's Day

DEC
- **01** World AIDS Day
- **03** International Day of Persons with Disabilities

As per 2021 Calendar

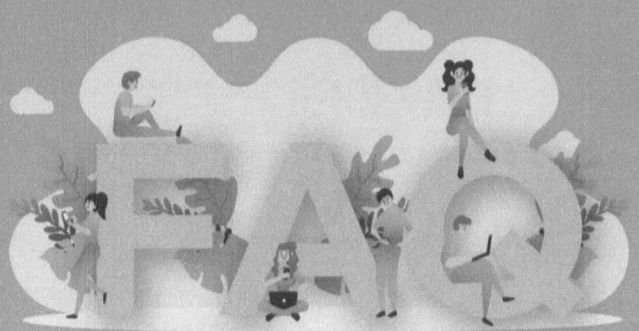

FAQs FOR PLANNING YOUR CAUSE BASED CAMPAIGN
PRE EVENT

Q. When to start the campaign ?

A. Start 1 week in advance preferably on a weekend.

Q. When it is advisable to conduct a camp if it is for a single day?

A. Preferably Sunday

Q. What is the ideal duration for a Campaign?

A. Short Campaigns can be for a day or two. Long Campaigns can be upto a month

Q. What are the communication essentials in a campaign?

A.
- Clear cut message on the nature of the campaign
- Resultant benefits of attending the camp
- Date/s & time of the campaign
- Venue of the campaign
- Contact Information
- Brand Logo + Association Partner Logos

Q. What Mediums can be used for promoting the campaign ?

A. Offline : TV Ads / Paper Ads / Hoardings / Bus Ads / Radio Ads / Wall Posters / Paper Inserts
Online : Google Adwords / Facebook Ads / Inside Brand Website promotion
Venue : Banners / Posters at your hospital

EVENT DAY

Q. What are the essential promo activities on the event day?

A.
- First, give a reminder message via sms / email / social media on the event day in the morning
- Use social media extensively. Apart from photos, take more videos and post it on the same day or use LIVE features in social media to get more mileage during the event
- Ask people who got benefited from the campaign to share their views Post Event

POST EVENT

Q. What should be the post event activity?

A. Share a thank you note covering the overall success of the campaign

7 STEPS INVOLVED IN
CAUSE BASED MARKETING CAMPAIGN

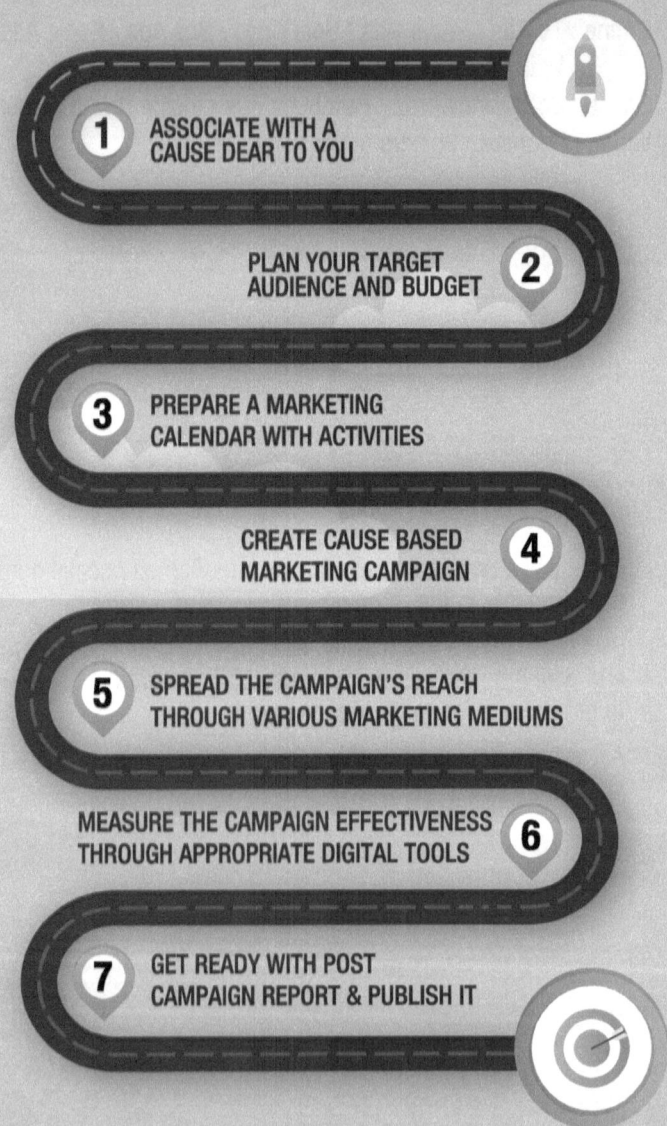

1. ASSOCIATE WITH A CAUSE DEAR TO YOU
2. PLAN YOUR TARGET AUDIENCE AND BUDGET
3. PREPARE A MARKETING CALENDAR WITH ACTIVITIES
4. CREATE CAUSE BASED MARKETING CAMPAIGN
5. SPREAD THE CAMPAIGN'S REACH THROUGH VARIOUS MARKETING MEDIUMS
6. MEASURE THE CAMPAIGN EFFECTIVENESS THROUGH APPROPRIATE DIGITAL TOOLS
7. GET READY WITH POST CAMPAIGN REPORT & PUBLISH IT

Note: Generally, Cause Based Campaigns should be long term and should have a 12months marketing action calendar plan with defined goals to arrive at measured outcomes. Given above is a single activity plan which can be used for all your cause based campaigns that can happen throughout the year with changes as required.

Nutrition Awareness Campaign

Apollo Hospitals conducted a 360 degree online & offline Nutrition Awareness Cause Campaign that spoke about nutritional goodness in natural food. They launched a booklet on the subject and gamified the experience by making people play the snake and ladder game with a twist - health foods took them up by ladders and junk food took them down with snakes.

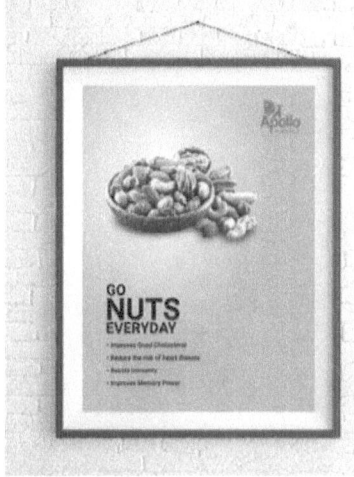
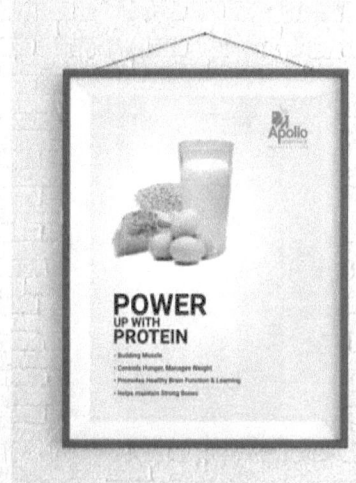

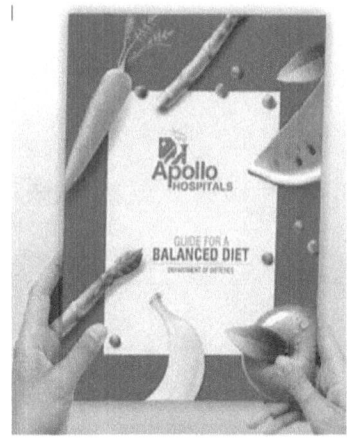

NUTRITION GAMES

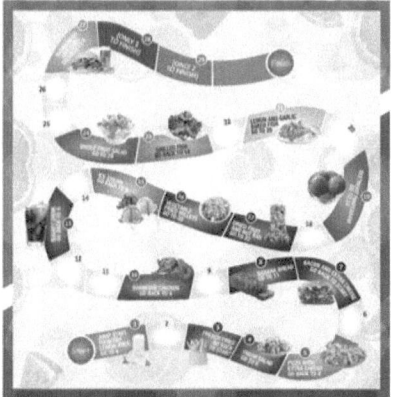

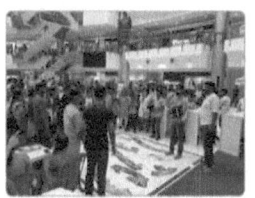
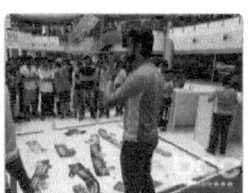

CASE STUDY

Breast Cancer Awareness by Carilion Clinic

Cause Campaign on Breast Cancer Awareness by Carilion Clinic. The clinic called the campaign "Yes ma'am" and hashtagged it with the same. Various activities and digital campaigns were flagged off as an off-shoot of the same. Later the hospital became one of the most trusted centers for mammography.

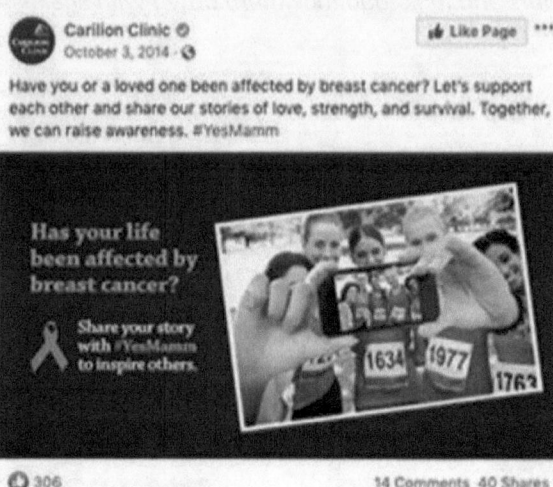

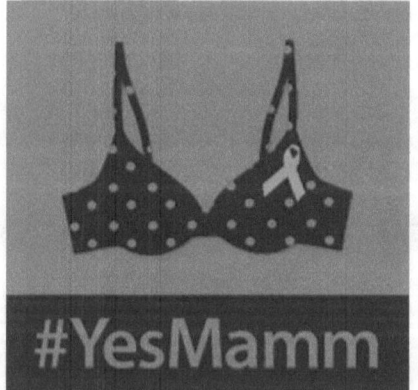

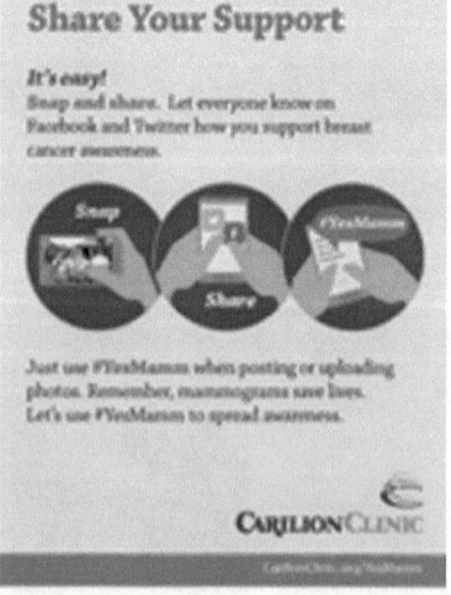

CASE STUDY

UnitedHealthcare Campaign: We Dare You

UnitedHealthcare created an interactive campaign in order to promote healthier habits. The campaign created monthly dares, quizzes, and prizes on its website. UnitedHealthcare worked on encouraging their followers to make one small healthy change per month and document it on social media.

The healthcare ads campaign was successful for many reasons. Followers of the media are responsive to challenges – it's fun, harmless, and spreads awareness.

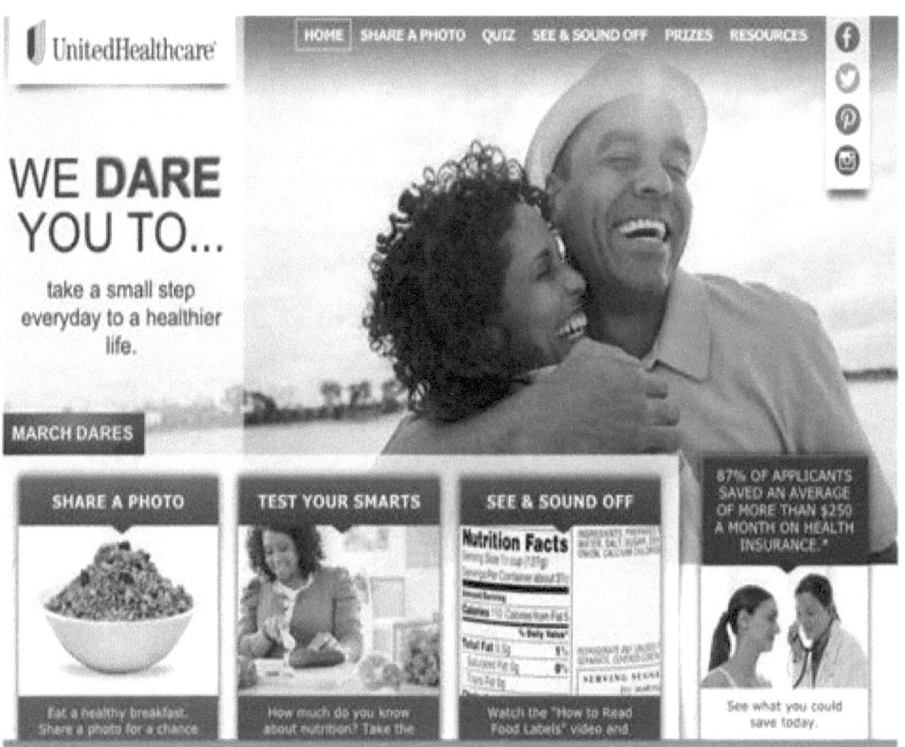

Ice Bucket Challenge

The Ice Bucket Challenge, sometimes called the ALS Ice Bucket Challenge, was an activity involving the dumping of a bucket of ice water over a person's head, either by another person or self-administered, to promote awareness of the disease amyotrophic lateral sclerosis and encourage donations to research.

CASE STUDY

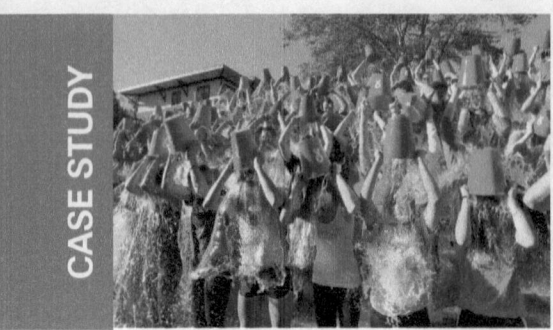

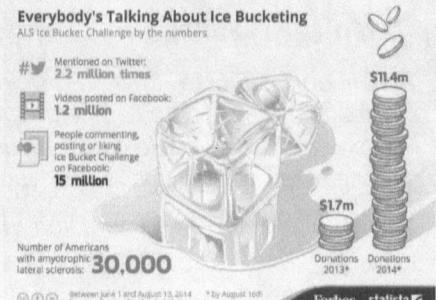

Everybody's Talking About Ice Bucketing
ALS Ice Bucket Challenge by the numbers

Mentioned on Twitter: **2.2 million times**
Videos posted on Facebook: **1.2 million**
People commenting, posting or liking Ice Bucket Challenge on Facebook: **15 million**
Number of Americans with amyotrophic lateral sclerosis: **30,000**

Donations 2013*: $1.7m
Donations 2014*: $11.4m

Between June 1 and August 13, 2014 * by August 16th
Sources: Twitter, Facebook, ALS Association

Forbes statista

CHALLENGE ME

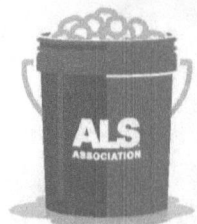

THE ALS ICE BUCKET CHALLENGE WAS A GLOBAL PHENOMENON THAT RAISED MILLIONS OF DOLLARS AND CHANGED THE FIGHT AGAINST ALS FOREVER.

DONATIONS RAISED THROUGH THE 2014 ALS ICE BUCKET CHALLENGE SPURRED A MASSIVE INCREASE IN THE ALS ASSOCIATION'S CAPACITY TO INVEST IN PROMISING RESEARCH, THE DEVELOPMENT OF ASSISTIVE TECHNOLOGIES, AND INCREASED ACCESS TO CARE AND SERVICES FOR PEOPLE WITH ALS.

5 NEW GENES discovered since the ALS Ice Bucket Challenge, which will spur new therapies.

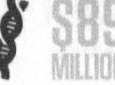 **$89 MILLION** committed to research to advance the search for treatments and a cure.

 MORE THAN TRIPLED our ALS research budget. The ALS Association is the largest private funder of research worldwide.

 15,000 PEOPLE per year helped with community-based services through their local ALS Association Chapter.

FIRST EVER guidance submitted to the FDA to speed the development & approval of new ALS treatments.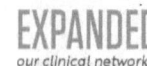

 **EXPANDED** our clinical network to increase availability of ALS care.

11 global research collaborations that have already resulted in 2 new antisense drugs targeting SOD1 and C9orf72 in development.

$115 MILLION donated through the ALS Ice Bucket Challenge during an 8 week period in 2014.

MORE THAN 17 MILLION people uploaded their challenge videos to Facebook.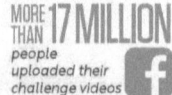

INVESTED in technology and innovation to help people with ALS live fuller lives.

THE ALS ICE BUCKET CHALLENGE DIRECTLY IMPACTED THE LIVES OF PEOPLE IN YOUR COMMUNITY:

 CLINICAL CARE   ASSISTIVE TECHNOLOGY   SUPPORT GROUPS

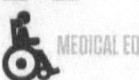 MEDICAL EQUIPMENT LOAN   CARE GRANTS 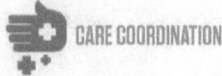 CARE COORDINATION

PARTICIPATE · ADVOCATE · DONATE

Learn more about the impact of the ALS Ice Bucket Challenge at ChallengeALS.org

© 2019 ALS Association

STRATEGY 2

"WHEN YOUR PRESENCE IS STRONGLY FELT, YOUR PURPOSE IS FAIRLY MET"

PERSONAL BRANDING

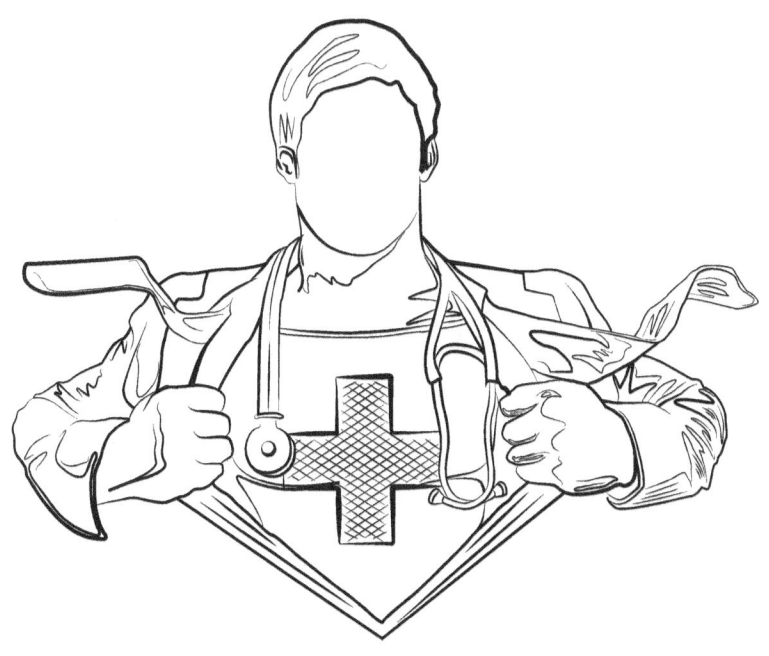

Brand ? Branding ??

When the whole world is talking about brands let us take some time out and answer the million-dollar question "what is a brand?" and "what is branding?"

A brand is a potent idea with a specific set of identities and a set of characteristics that are unique to itself. A brand can be a product, service, person, ideology or a mere thing.

Branding is a structured process of positioning and popularizing the key brand message to its desired set of target audiences through a well-defined strategy so that a desirable impression about the brand gets formed.

Now think about all those products, service providers and people you think are brands. Now ponder over how they have become brands that they are today.

If any person can become a brand then what is "personal branding"?

Personal branding is the process of crafting one's identity in the minds of people as it is desired to be. The identity has to be taken from the core of the individual's belief system so the person becomes more relatable, desirable and trust-worthy. There has to be a perfect marriage between what he/she is and what he/she stands for to create a powerful personal brand.

Personal branding for doctors

Personal branding for a doctor is through their unique personal merit, style of practice, what difference they bring on to their consultation tables and how different they make it reach.

All that a doctor needs to become a personal brand is that factor of originality connected with their core value system. Originality builds trust, attracts attention and the right kind of relationships to help you reach your professional goals. This immensely powerful trait of originality, when used for noble acts like standing up for a mission, can deeply root one's identity in the same desirable market.

A personal brand of a doctor will be more of a rooted impression than just any other doctor looking to leave a positive impact through awareness communication. Taking the initiative to build a personal brand will bind each outreach activity that you have done to reinforce that one powerful message that you stand for.

The one powerful message is the mission of your life, every activity that you perform to achieve the noble mission is actually of enacting your personal brand. A personal brand is not a forceful identity or a fake entity; it is about living your true self and communicating consciously to your surroundings so that your noble mission is achieved through the support of your personal brand audience. The act of personal branding can motivate your audience to achieve high ideals in life like yours by taking you as their inspiration.

8 Commandments of Personal branding

1. Get known to the world by your name

Your name becomes your address. By just making people remember your name makes them remember you for your practice, the whole existence of you as a brand is established. As the purpose of personal branding is to consciously make people remember you for your expertise and other allied qualities straight through your name than any other related identity.

The whole world searches for you by remembering your name when you are a personal brand. Your videos, website, and social media profiles are all keyed in with your exact name on how you use it with proper consistent syntax. You will be known with your name and not sub-identities when you establish a personal brand.

Introduce your practice to the whole world, imprint it with your image. Your personal brand will introduce you to a whole new set of audience collective containing a mixed set of prospects. The very technique of personal branding aims to not just popularize you but to sculpt a long-lasting impression of you with a well-molded purpose attached to it.

2. There is a difference between a well-known doctor and a preferred doctor, become both

Personal branding takes you to more number of prospects, once you kick start your personal branding journey people will get to know you better. The more they know, the more you will win their trust and preference. Winning trust is not just about converting them as your patients but, it is about becoming that sole source they would look up to when it comes to any health issue they want advice for that particular area of your expertise. Imagine people recognizing you from elsewhere without even meeting you for once but connecting with you for what you stand for.

Understand that familiarity alone doesn't breed success; ultimately what matters is whether they are preferred in the market. Many well-known doctors who have become personal brands through diligent PR and public speaking might not be real-time preferred doctors and out of the ones who are busy in practice might not be that great at traits that are required to be well known.

Also, if you are on one part of the extreme there are good chances for you to attract new patients but sustaining the momentum is greatly questionable if you don't really deliver on your promise.

The ultimate goal of creating a personal brand that one wants to become will organically be reached when one understands the difference between these two- "preferred" and "well-known". By harnessing the best practices in becoming the well known and working one's own strengths will promise the personal brand a rapid increase in preference.

3 Feed your personas with your personality

A persona is a representation of a collective group of prospects with similar characteristics created to understand and categorize the type of people your personal brand attracts.

Your personas want to know you for who you are, your style of practice and your current whereabouts. They want to know how you make your patients feel, so feed your daily activities and get across your real lively personality to them. Let the best of both worlds- online and offline bring you closer to your personas.

Take enough steps to track and analyze the trend of in-flowing patients and crack a set pattern. Every aspect of the patient reaching you can mean a different impact factor for your personal brand so, know what they are reaching you for, when and why. With this, you can analyze your practice's strengths and weakness for instance they may reach you for your deep consultation, the effectiveness of your patient coordinators, proximity, infrastructure or a combination of these. These factors are mere extensions of your personal brand, people connect to your intangible personal brand through these tangible factors. Know what they are choosing you for, to deliver better care to your patients and grow your practice manifolds.

4 Establish a personal connect

The biggest challenge of attaining patient satisfaction today is that patients aren't able to spend quality time with their doctors explaining their concerns which is a common complaint. Personal connect helps you to establish a deep bond with your patients and help them experience your personal brand's message directly through the source so establish personal connect through 1-1 consultation, hear them, give them the time they need and comfort them . In such circumstances, it only happens that the patients become effective brand advocates.

The personal connection will satisfy your patients and will strengthen your practice. The most personal you can get to one is to be handed over the responsibility of taking care of one's well being. So, when you are given the highest form of responsibility hold on to the strong bond that comforts and gives confidence to your patients.

Remember that little things matter. To your patients, every act of concern is a great deal. Through your personal branding channels, it is only natural that you will invite many real-time potential patient engagements, make sure you reply your best to each one of them. Look to etch the significance of your effort at every point.

5. Be ambitious about a patient support community, not just a follower base

Don't just look to create a conglomerate of people who may need your service, address the affected community at large and become their factor of solace, hope, and guidance. Make a significant difference in the whole world of your specialty. Look to help people in their journeys of cure, instruct on any doubts a patient may have and promote healthy living in general.

Patients need periodic help and not just a set of consultations/planned procedures. Continuous support from you as a personal brand will make you win a secure place in a patient's mind and heart. A patient support community can be created through effective usage of personalised online platforms or even open ones like Facebook groups or Youtube channels where you can address queries efficiently. When poeple who are affected with similar ailments get your message and experience the tangible difference it can make in aligning their life towards good health, they will become your brand advocates and spread your message faster to the ones who have similar ailments.

6. An individual scores more than an institute

Realize that people want to be proud of their doctor and any brand will gain credibility only through the individual who directly serves the patient. Patients see you as the source of their satisfying healthcare experience and then the healthcare brand involved. Even an established brand needs a doctor who commands his own place in a patient's heart.

There is a sea of difference between just a doctor and a conscious personal brand, and what value each of them will bring to the organization. A personal brand can demand everything a luxurious practice demands, as he/she will be one of those factors who keep the patients flowing in.

The advantage of having a personal brand inside a big organizational brand is that they have their own advantage in terms of revenue, value, added familiarity, social media traffic, PR element, and patient's preference.

7. Don't get shadowed, glow and grow in your own light

As a successful practitioner you may be practicing for a healthcare brand that probably has more recall factors among your potential patient base, don't get underwhelmed.

Understand that there is no age limit to peer pressure. In your context the actual peer pressure is how relatively successful your senior professionals & co-practitioners are and how the immediate industry around you is growing rapidly. Don't get overwhelmed by what is going on around you, as you will lose your way if you follow theirs. Instead, find your own way, your own style and your own formula of uncovering your true path of glory and light.

Even if you work for a big brand you will have your own set of skills to offer. When you are a personal brand in a big corporate hospital you will take the pedestal without any extra efforts. There is no denial about the fact that people will come in search of you with no alternative identities but directly your address- Your name!

8. Be a forerunner, not a chaser

Being a chaser will land you up anywhere but where you really want to go, so be a forerunner. By being a forerunner you set the tone, standards and you show the way for the rest of others in your fraternity to follow.

Everyday Healthcare is undergoing enormous changes in creating patient-centric systems, try to learn and show others the way to get benefit out of it. By being the forerunner you really become the first in that area of expertise.

Ethical Hospital Branding & Marketing

There are different aspects of personal branding in healthcare that the world around you is still hesitating to dive in and explore. The hesitation is a mere result of "Will I be going overboard?" Now the very fact that you are the first one to take up a technique of personal branding in your own known circle and implementing it in your strategy means you are way ahead in accelerating the reach of your practice and this seldom does count for "going overboard" if you very well play within the rules of healthcare branding and marketing. So, stop waiting for somebody to pass the relay torch to you and instead take the first leap all by yourself to enjoy the benefits of a personal brand in leaps and bounds.

Personal branding is the one and only powerful way to navigate through the chaotic situation in these turbulent times and build your practice without much trouble. Build your personal brand through ways you will be really proud of. Don't curb the fullest power of the powerful message of what you want to tell the world. Even in the most daunting times stand up for what you are really meant to stand up for. Be known for that one thing the world will respect you and revere you for eternity. Build your personal brand! Build your legacy!

2
PERSONAL BRANDING
ACTION PLAN

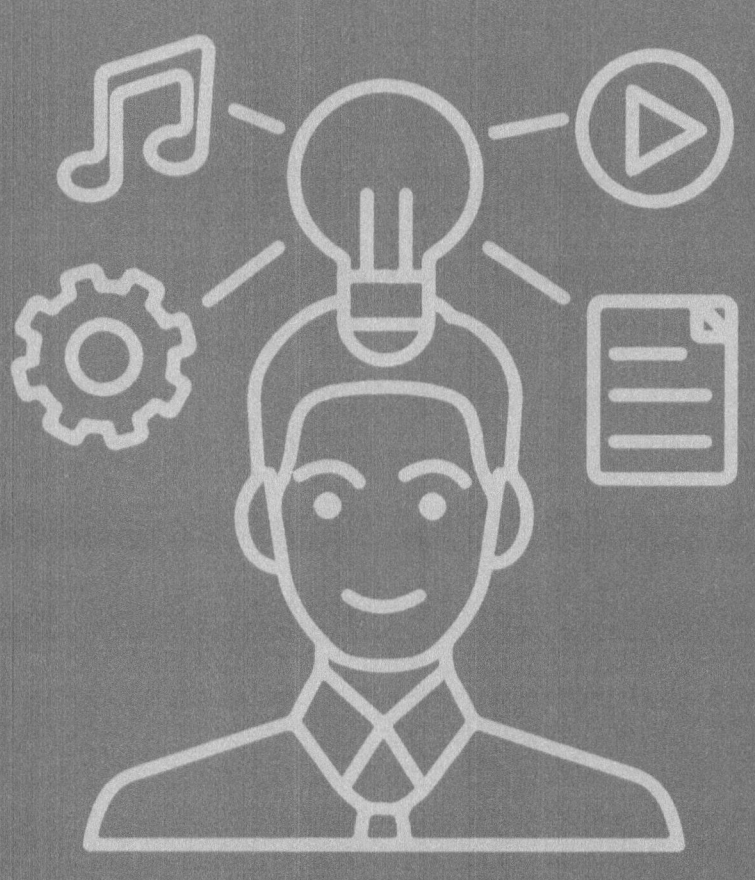

PERSONAL BRANDING FOR DOCTORS
CHECKLIST (1/5)

CASE STUDY

		Yes	No
1	Have you compiled a Book of case studies?	☐	☐
2	Is each case study narrated in story form and with medical terminologies (which will be used for narrating to the public and fraternity)?	☐	☐
3	Have you published your case studies in Online Forums / Private Groups / your Website / Journals?	☐	☐
4	Have you presented your case studies in CMEs?	☐	☐

PROFILE

1	Have you covered Key Milestones in a snapshot (One important thing that will position you rightly in their mind has to be captured)?	☐	☐
2	Have you made your profile with Achievements & Accomplishment listed in Chronological Order?	☐	☐

8 STEPS FOR PERSONAL BRANDING

PASS YOUR LEGACY
(Opportunities will chase your organisation looking at your good works and will help in your organisation brand development)

MAKE YOUR DIRECT COMMUNICATION CHANNELS OPEN
(Be accessible to people via whatsapp / chat / mail / helpline / on appointment)

KEEP BUILDING YOUR AUDIENCE
(Be sincere & consistent in your good works)

START WITH ONE ACTIVITY & YOU WILL GET MANY
(People observing you will open up other opportunities, grab them)

PLAN A SERIES OF CAUSE BASED ACTIVITIES
(Camps /Awareness Videos in Youtube & FB / Talk Shows / Local Meet Ups / Local PR)

KEEP YOUR PROFILE UPDATED & VISIBLE ONLINE & OFFLINE
(People will want to know more about you once you reach them. This will open up possibilities for various collaborations)

MARRY YOUR MISSION WITH YOUR CAUSE & SPECIALTY
(Pick a cause dear to your specialty)

DEFINE YOUR MISSION IN LIFE
(This will define who you are to the world & what you stand for)

Note : Utmost sincerity and honesty is required in building your brand. Helping people genuinely should be the objective, by doing so people will help your organisation brand.

PERSONAL BRANDING FOR DOCTORS CHECKLIST

		Yes	No
3	Does your Achievements & Accomplishments cover the following		
A	Academic	☐	☐
B	Worked under some renowned name	☐	☐
C	Published Research Papers	☐	☐
D	Articles Published in Leading Journals	☐	☐
E	Awards & Accolades	☐	☐
F	Practice Achievements	☐	☐
G	Key Cases Attended	☐	☐
H	Hands-on training with a renowned trainer	☐	☐
4	Do you have your profile handy in both hard copy and soft copy?	☐	☐
5	Is your profile available online?	☐	☐

COMMUNICATION TOUCH POINTS

		Yes	No
1	Are you easy to find online?	☐	☐
2	Do you have a website in your name?	☐	☐
3	Do you have a dedicated phone number to reach you?	☐	☐

PERSONAL BRANDING FOR DOCTORS CHECKLIST (3/5) Yes No

		Yes	No
4	Do you have a dedicated email id to reach you?	☐	☐
5	Are you active in Social Media like FB, Twitter & Insta? (even one medium is fine)	☐	☐
6	Do you respond to queries people post via online mediums?	☐	☐
7	Are you good with handling FB Messenger?	☐	☐
8	Are you active in Whatsapp?	☐	☐

CAUSE

		Yes	No
1	Have you involved yourself in cause based campaigns on your own or supported any organisation?	☐	☐
2	Was the cause campaign related to your specialty?	☐	☐
3	Have you identified a cause to associate with?	☐	☐
4	Do you know how to conduct a cause based campaign?	☐	☐
5	Does your mission in life synchronise with your cause?	☐	☐
6	Are you determined to influence others to take up a cause and inspire others?	☐	☐

AWARENESS EDUCATION

                                                                    Yes   No

1. Did you conduct any awareness education program?   ☐   ☐

2. Have you written any health awareness articles / blogs
   which got published in any newspaper / journal / website?   ☐   ☐

3. Have you created educational youtube videos
   relating to your specialty?   ☐   ☐

4. Have you created videos answering questions which are
   frequently asked by people like myth busters?   ☐   ☐

5. Do you have awareness posters/ leaflets
   at your practice place?   ☐   ☐

TESTIMONIES

1. Have you got testimonies from your patients in
   text / video form?   ☐   ☐

2. Do you have a collection of all your testimonies ?   ☐   ☐

3. Are your testimonies published with your patient
   permission online/offline ?   ☐   ☐

4. Are the patient testimonies visible in your practice place?   ☐   ☐

PERSONAL BRANDING FOR DOCTORS CHECKLIST (5/5)

BRAND AUDIENCE

Yes   No

1. Is your brand audience growing everyday? ☐ ☐

2. Are you effectively measuring their growth? ☐ ☐

3. Are you creating the content they like? ☐ ☐

4. Do you get a pulse of what they are looking forward to? ☐ ☐

5. Are you consistent in posting your content? ☐ ☐

SWOT ANALYSIS

STRENGTHS 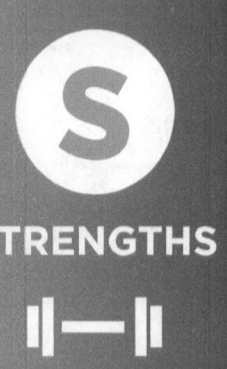	**WEAKNESS** 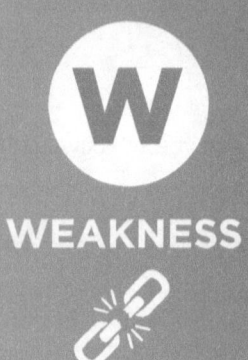
OPPORTUNITIES 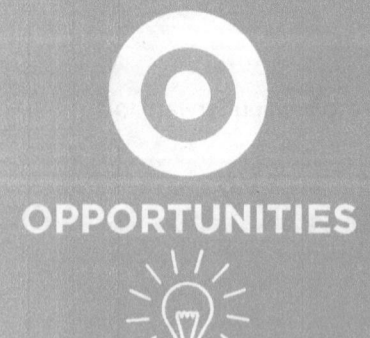	**THREATS** 

STRENGTHS

Enumerate your strong points

1 What type of work do you want to accelerate doing?

2 When you are working in a team what is it that your are praised for the most?

3 What is that one purpose that excites you about your practice and motivates you to reach more people?

4 What is the strong emotion behind your passionate activity?

5 How can your strong emotions help you to achieve your final goal?

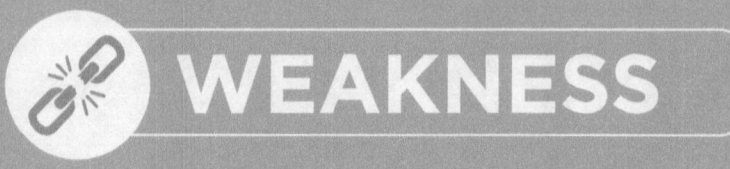

WEAKNESS

Enumerate your weakness

1 What are the weaknesses that stand between you and your goal?

2 Is aligning your team to your goals a big challenge you often face?

3 Are you concentrating too much on your daily engagements?

4 Do you ignore your negative feedback?

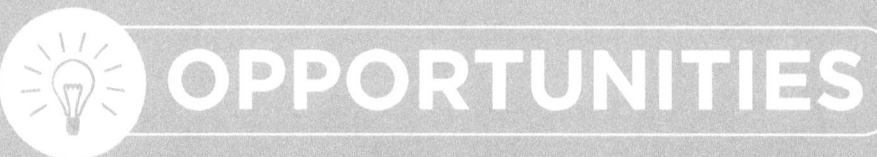

OPPORTUNITIES

Enumerate your Opportunities

1 How far do you want to reach with your marketing goals?

2 Are you looking to partner with right people who can help you achieve your goals?

3 Are you looking to associate with the right organizations who can take you closer to your dreams?

4 Are you considering upskilling in areas there is a big demand now and in the near future?

5. Are you considering tech up-gradaton to accelerate your workflow?

6. Are you looking at right collaboration to scale up faster

7. Are you looking at innovative collaboration models which can provide easy growth?

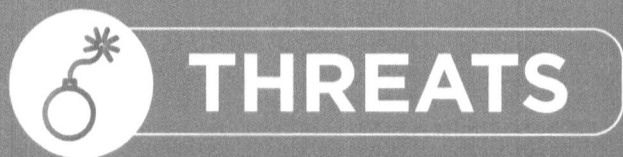

THREATS

Enumerate your Threats

1. Do you lack big time on mandatory skills and efforts?

2. Do you see your patient satisfaction levels going down the hill?

3. Is your patient count declining?

4. Do you see nascent brands growing at an unmatchable pace compared to yours?

5. Are you fearing stagnation or irrelevance to current patients?

6. Are you struggling to be digitally savvy to meet your patient's digital demands?

Note

STRATEGY 3

"A MAN WITHOUT A FACE IS THE SAME AS A BRAND WITHOUT A LOGO"

LOGO DESIGN & POSITIONING

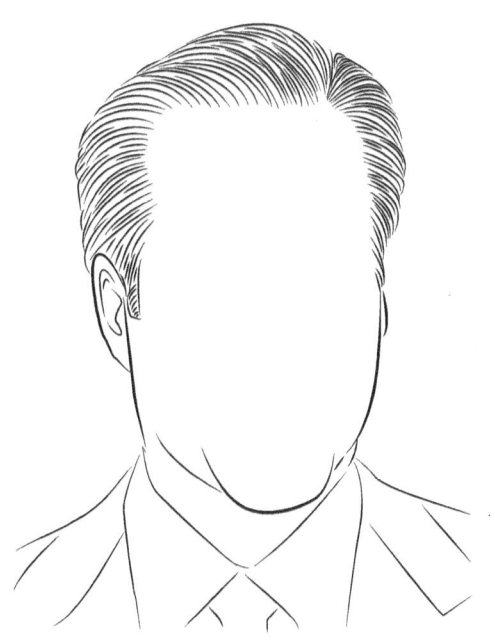

The face of your brand

Your hospital brand logo is the most powerful identity that helps you get identified among your brand audience. This is the most powerful imagery of your organisation, so, take great care in crafting it well. It should truly reflect what your brand stands for. Once the logo is defined that becomes the face of your brand and whenever they think about your brand - your brand logo comes into their mind. Once you define it and make it synonymous with your brand, then people will start recognizing your brand by the presence of your logo. We are living in a world where we see people are increasingly deciding to opt services of a brand by the mere look of it.

Make sure you craft your logo well so that it synchronizes well with your value system, which becomes evident for the beholders. A logo that appears in various brand collaterals, like a badge that is worn by employees with pride, adds significant meaning to their life. So, it is not something that needs to be taken lightly but with utmost involvement as it is the face of your brand. A brand need not look big or small by the mere look of it. Even a small brand can look big when it is next to the giants by the mere look of it, if it is designed and positioned well.

10 Commandments of Hospital Logo Design

1 Do not Look like Others

Don't go with logo makers that carry predefined templates to represent who you are, which will ultimately carve a face for your brand, same as others. Make sure you take enough internal meetings or brainstorming sessions to fully encapsulate how your brand personality should look like. People will take very few seconds to understand whether they are dealing with a professional brand or not, by the mere look of your logo. With more original thinking that suits your brand style evolve a unique brief that will give birth to a logo that is truly meant to be yours and yours only.

2 Do not Copy Others

You can get inspiration by looking at some of the logos of brand leaders but copying is a heinous crime, which not only gets you sued for intellectual copyright violation but also you will bury your originality and reputation. By trying to look like others is also no good. If your brand is really good - then the brand from where you have copied the looks of your logo enjoys the fruits and on the other side, if that brand earns bad reputation later, without any fault of yours, you will also get into trouble.

3. Be Original. Be You

Everyone in this world is a real masterpiece and God made us that way. If we dig a little deeper into our capabilities and the way how we serve patients, we can find a unique system which is at place, working for us well. And that is the system which is truly ours. The brand DNA is made out of it. Whether you communicate this or not, that closed set of audience who approach you will keep coming to you for the that system. The system ingrained in your Brand DNA is Unique and is a Great Success which needs instant communication to the world. Those values, if ingrained in the logo can make your brand logo truly original. The world will appreciate your original self more than the copied version. And by being original you set new standards.

4. Be Bold & find your audience

Boldness in taking a stand will set you apart from others and also you will carve a new path to success through your approach. The clarity in presenting your thoughts will go a long way in attracting the right audience that your brand is meant to serve. Make sure boldness & clarity becomes the essential ingredients in your brand logo. Choose fonts that are bold and clear from a distance. People may get less than 3 seconds to take in any message on the go and if your logo is the message, make sure you deliver it well. The fonts you use and the symbols in your brand logo are the exact depictions of the values you stand for. When there is clarity, there is familiarity and familiarity breeds success.

5. Avoid Complicated Symbols

Make sure the symbolism in your logo conveys very clearly what you stand for and avoid ambiguous and unclear symbolism. The symbolism has to be an extension of your value system at practice. Generally, symbols can exhibit features like care, empathy, support, strength in their medical specialty, specialty-specific symbols, medical excellence, etc. Apart from this you can also have the acronyms of your brand also as a symbol. Some symbols become more memorable than others and simplicity plays a vital role here. Ingraining simplicity in your symbols will help in the effective reproduction of the logo on any medium/surface.

6. Say "NO" to thin fonts & very long brand names

Avoid using thin fonts as it will cause a catastrophic effect on brand readability. Yes, logos have to be clearly readable. It's advisable to maintain fonts that are easy to read from a distance so that the brand name stands out clearly. Avoid using long-form registered names of the brand, instead, use acronyms or the main brand name removing the prefixes and suffixes. It's an important point to note-when your logo takes lesser space to represent your brand, clearly that's how effective it becomes. Remove "Ltd", "LLP" in the suffixes as they are only for statutory purposes.

7. Do not use multiple colours

Avoid using more than 2 colours in the logo. The best is a single color and also in some cases, 2 colors would do well. In rare cases, where the subject demands; then go for multi-colors. Single/dual coloured logos look neat and graceful looking. With lesser colors, comes lesser spending, when you are trying for a special type of printing. Also, lesser colours mean lesser clutter, when you design your brand stationery with this limited one / two color formula your brand stands out from the rest in the category. Everything starting from your signage, badge, biz card, letterhead, etc will seem to create profound brand presence.

8 Make sure your logo is easily reproducible

When your logo is simple, it can be reproduced easily on any surface like glass, cloth embroidery ...etc without losing its integrity. This saves the confusion whether it is the same logo or not. Design a logo with the end output in mind so that your logo will not miss out on any essential feature that it needs to carry and maintain its utmost integrity.

9 Maintain Harmony

We find some logos completely disharmonious, whether it be the colours they choose, the proportion in which the alignment is made, fonts chosen/made or the entire composition in which the symbol, font, and colours appear. Make sure you maintain the utmost harmony in your symbol, font, and colours you choose to maintain the utmost impact. Harmonious logos look very professional and cultured and that's the feeling people will get about your brand the moment they see it. When there is harmony in the logo it tells a lot about your healthcare brand, every time.

10 Deeper Meaning

Even simple looking logos can have much deeper meanings or layers of communication. It can be understood/interpreted based on the audience. It is good to have deeper meanings embedded in the logo so that it looks ageless and strong over the years. The meaning again can be derived from the acronyms, values, your inspiration, your future dream, aspirations, etc. Always have futuristic elements ingrained in your logo, after all, a brand is made to sustain and thrive for generations together. And when you handover this brand to the next generation, they should also want to retain the ageless values intact and each time when they look at the logo it should remind them about those high principles which you made it stand for.

Brand Positioning

Positioning plays an important role as it tells the world the mission of the brand, it tells the world what problem this brand is set to solve or why this brand is more desirable and bound to aspire you. The value system/mission can be presented well in words with the help of the right positioning line. When the positioning is strong people get the message directly as to what the brand is bound to do.

Arriving at the right positioning line which matches your brand DNA is very crucial as this is the line that will be read by a lot many to understand your brand's purpose. Let us look at various ways to arrive at your brand positioning. The positioning can be based on medical excellence, leadership, tech-driven, values-driven, specialty-specific, recovery & happy life, friendly & family-like care, etc. Pick a positioning that suits and reflects your brand better.

Brand Positioning can be established through various campaigns that the brand is carrying forward to promote a cause. Positioning does not only comprise of a tagline but also brings in a wold of clarity in so many aspects. In every campaign, the positioning becomes the guiding principle, the positioning defines the tonality of the campaign, the type of campaigns the brand will undertake to reach its desired audience, the mediums that the brand will take to reach the campaign, for what the campaigns will be made, how the internal communication guidelines will be framed and so on. Brand positioning is not just a statement, it is a governing law of your brand that guides precisely every brand communication activity of your brand.

With the right brand logo and effective positioning, your brand can become an integral part of the fraternity.

3
BRAND LOGO POSITIONING
ACTION PLAN

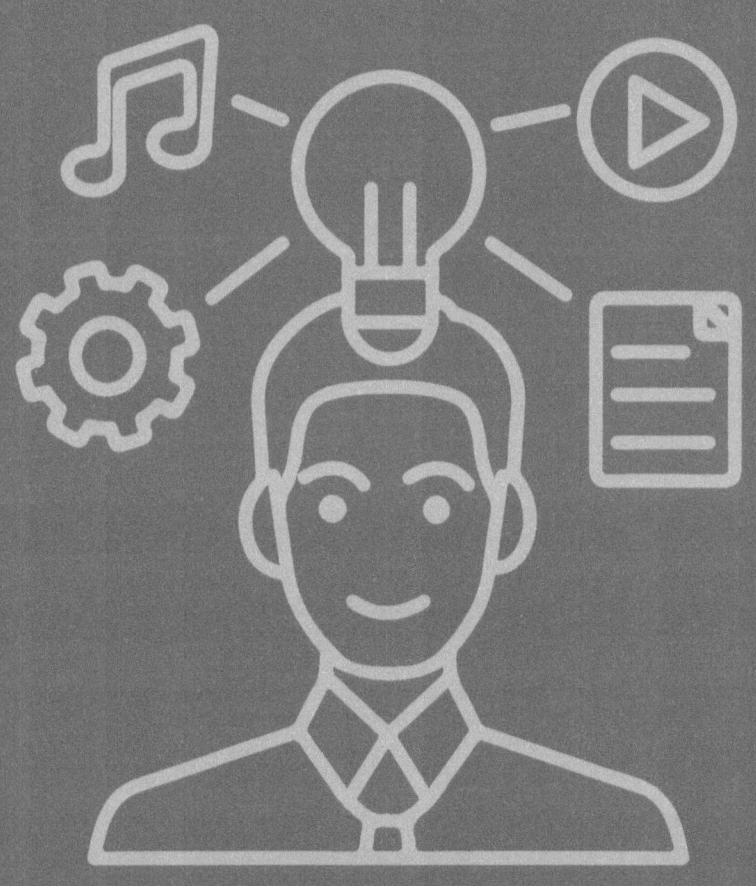

How to design your Hospital Logo ?

3 STEP

BLUEPRINT TO CREATE YOUR HOSPITAL LOGO

FONT 01
COLOR 02
SYMBOL 03

CHOOSE YOUR FONT

A
Perfect Bold font you can also choose to create your own font.

B
Make sure your brand name is readable.

C
Choose a balanced font. Fonts like heventica, coolgoose, harabara..etc are in this category and you can explore more

D
Make sure the fonts dont have sharp edges - they can be flat or soft

---

CHOOSE YOUR COLOR

A
Choose colours which are soft, smooth & pleasing

B
Some widely used brand colours and their significance.

Blue : Transparency, Professionalism
Turquoise : Peace, Control
Yellow : Approachable, Friendly
Orange : Warmth, Freedom
Green : Calmness, Balance
Pink : Love, Nurturing

C
You can choose the color of your choice as long as it matches with your brand DNA

CREATE YOUR SYMBOL

A
Create an unique symbol that represents what you stand for

B
Make sure the symbol is simple and easy to reproduce

C
It can have deeper hidden meanings but with one obvious meaning to the target audience

D
Make a balanced composition of font, color and symbol to get your logo ready

3C TEST
FOR YOUR LOGO

CLARITY | CONSISTENCY | CONNECT

If you already have a logo made, make your logo pass this test.

Does your logo pass this 3C test?

1. Clarity Test

1 (a). Is your logo clearly readable from a distance?

1 (b). Is your logo single colored or dual colored?

2. Consistency Test

2 (a). Is there a guideline for your logo to follow, when it appears in various formats?

2 (b). Is your logo consistent when it gets reproduced in stationery, uniform or signage?

3. Connect Test

3 (a). Does your logo carry meaningful symbolism that your brand stands for?

3 (b). Can your target audience relate to the visual symbolism your logo carries?

Note :
Desirable answer for the above is : **'Yes'**. It means your logo has passed 3C Test. If **'No'** then align your logo well as per the above test

How to brief your agency on logo design?
(Fill this format and send it to your creative agency)

1 Full Name of your Organisation

2 Brand Name

3 Preferred Colours (if any & why)

4 Preferred Fonts (if any & why)

5 Preferred Symbols (if any & why)

6 How according to you, your dream logo should look like

| 7 | What are your brand attributes? What does your brand stand for ? Share your Vision / Mission Statements |

| 8 | Which are the 3 International & National Brand Logos you aspire & why (any business category) |

| 9 | Which are the 3 International Brand Logos you aspire & why (in your category) |

| 10 | Which are the 3 National Brand Logos you aspire & why (in your category) |

| 11 | What to avoid in your logo |

| 12 | Any specific Comments |

To Rule the World, Define a Rule.

Branding your organisation helps you define your value system you practise and the value you can deliver.

Brand Identity / Logo is the visual representation of your brand personality it tells a lot about your brand with the right combination of visual symbolisms, typography, colours and composition.

Brand Identity Manual Snippets

Logo Rationale

The bold look is given by this customised font which makes the brand stand out clearly well.

The symbolism of bone in the letter "i" represents the category of business elegantly well.

The resultant benefit of availing the brand service is illustrated through the symbolism of a human who is now relieved from pain, feels relaxed, almost feels like flying in air.

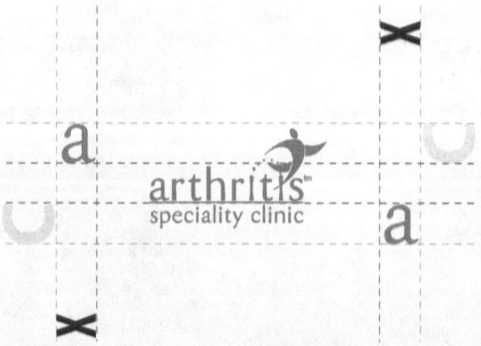

Taking "X" as the height of the character 'S' in the logo type, the exclusion zone would be the area defined by leaving a uniform margin "X" units on all four sides.

Implementing the brand colors across media

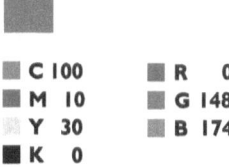

- C 100
- M 10
- Y 30
- K 0

- R 0
- G 148
- B 174

Logo Versions

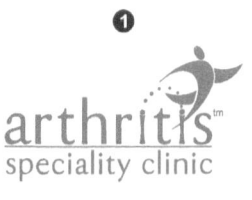

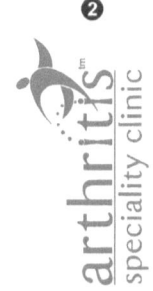

1. Standard Horizontal stacked arrangement
2. Vertical

Logo in Reverse

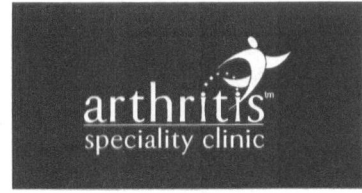

Premitted reverse version of the logo

The logo can be reversed out of either Black of 90% Gray or White on Gray (Original color of Logo). It should not be reversed out of an any other color. The sequence of colors should not be modified in any manner.

Typical Applications
External signage, environmental graphics, advertisements etc.

Scaling the logo

Max: Any desired size

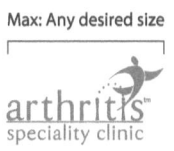

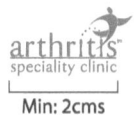

Min: 2cms

How to arrive at your positioning

5 Elements for Hospital Positioning

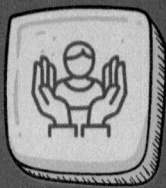
CARE — 01
It covers positioning pertaining to empathy, love, respect, concern

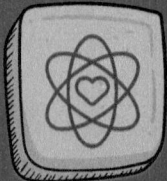
VALUES — 02
It covers positioning pertaining to transparency, ethics, human value

EXCELLENCE — 03
It covers positioning pertaining to longevity, quality standards, technical merit, experts, research

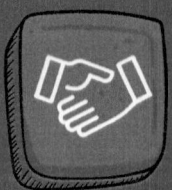
PROMISE — 04
It covers positioning pertaining to you will be well, delivery

TRUST — 05
(It covers positioning pertaining to longevity, excellence, delivery)

STRATEGY 4

"YOUR NETWORK IS YOUR NET WORTH"

WORD-OF-MOUTH MARKETING

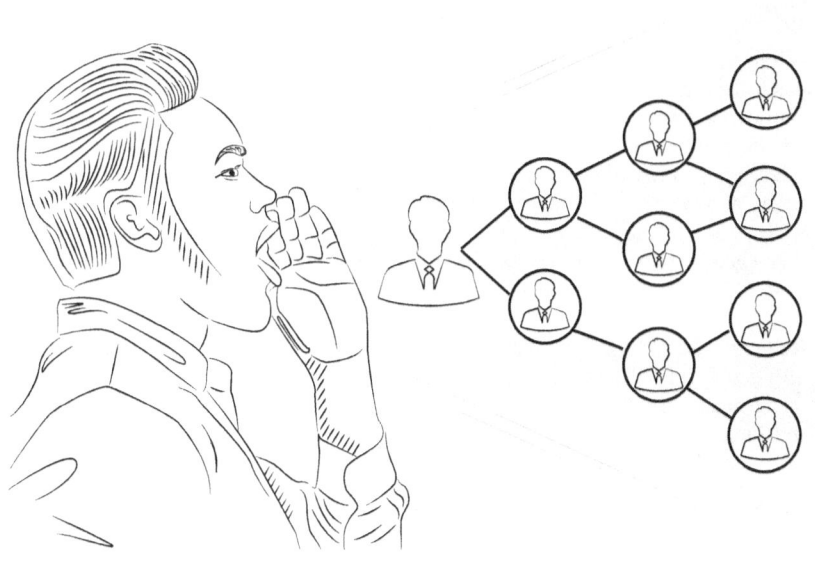

Have you ever sat down and analyzed-what got you the most number of patients even without intentional marketing?

You have successfully been getting patients so far. How do you think you have achieved that? It is through the ones who share a great relationship with your healthcare brand. These relationships have been loyal in growing your healthcare brand even when you didn't ask for it. People are anyway going to refer you for your expertise and great service by communicating to their own known contacts when they need a healthcare service. This is called word-of-mouth marketing.

Without you initiating word-of-mouth marketing for your healthcare brand, it is working for you and escalating your brand presence than any other strategy. If it can work so well with no invested efforts from your side then think about the same method of marketing with a more structured system from your side- it will grow your healthcare brand to miraculous heights.

This is possible through a practical, actionable, result-oriented strategy with referral marketing in mind. Have a structured referral marketing plan in place to drive the word-of-mouth factor in all the right directions without leakages, so you don't let your healthcare brand lose out. Give your referrers more inputs and more joy in being your active referral partner, the association will naturally become more functional and vital to your healthcare brand.

When your healthcare brand builds the right relationships with people and has built a network channel for itself through all the right ways then, there cannot be a substitute to this for landing your healthcare brand to serve all the right needs. When people like you more, they do you a favor by referring you to others and that's inherent human nature. So, when you tell your referral partners how much they mean to you they will start to bond with your healthcare brand more. Getting more close to people and getting these people closer to your healthcare brand by being mutually caring is the base of building a great referral marketing program.

Referral Marketing is the type of marketing that leverages one's network and builds it further. In healthcare, referral marketing can work with utmost dynamism with the right result-oriented approach and rightly anchored marketing strategy.

9 Commandments of Referral Marketing

1 Build a 4D referral plan to thrive, not just to survive

Utilize the dynamism of referral marketing to see prospects that may result in different benefits. 4D - Four Dimensions of referral marketing- Patient-to-Patient referral, Doctor-to-Doctor referral, Doctor-to-Patient referral, and Employee-to-Patient referral program.

Patient-to-Patient Referrals: When your patients love your service, they also love to pass on the message of your existence to the ones whom they know are in need of you. Patients are usually more than happy to be helping them in making the right healthcare decision. So make sure you realize the effectiveness of this mechanism of patients becoming your referral givers and concentrate on making your brand-patient relationship more perfect & happening.

Doctor-to-Patient Referrals: When Doctors in your circle have an immense level of trust in you, in the area of your specialization, they refer their patients to you hoping to get specialized care. So make sure all the Doctor to Patient referrals are handled with utmost care and keep the doctor who referred informed about the patient at every cruicial step - they will expect this from you. This is a very powerful chain in the WoM (Word of mouth) system and can get you a steady stream of referrals regularly in large numbers.

Doctor-to-Doctor Referrals: When you are in need of specialized hands in areas that compliment your specialization, you look out for reliable names in your close circle. And such names are referred by doctors whom you trust and who trust you. When the brand has to grow big it requires efforts of specialized hands coming together and that's where D-to-D referrals play a vital role.

Employee-to-Patient Referrals: Employees working for your healthcare brand make the best reliable source the public gets to interact with. So, when they pass on information about your healthcare brand as a solution to those in need, there is an instant investment of trust from the patient as they get to hear from those who live the brand. Make sure your organizational culture itself is in a way that promotes your employees as brand ambassadors.

2. Unleash your referral network's fullest potential by unleashing your fullest potential to them

Your referrers have to know you well for them to refer you to the kind of patients you will be able to help the most. They have to know your key specialty, specific strength to become your best referral partner.

To see the fruits of a referral marketing program you'll have to connect to your potential referrers and present referrers by constantly updating them about your capabilities and services and how your service has proved to be significant.

3. Give each referrer the ultimate reason to refer you

Every referrer refers to you for a reason that they think you befit or serve the best to your patients, which may not be known to you. But if you have to increase the impact of WoM on your practice then it is possible only by knowing the reason behind referral you have gained and analyzing them over a period of time.

This indeed will give you more clarity over your areas of strengths and areas you need to improve to deliver better care as a healthcare provider. Also, learn what can make you more preferred by your referral partners which can help you in understanding if you have to build on your competencies/

new-skill sets, improve staff training, add new capability or new equipment addition in your infrastructure.

4. Not amplifying the reach of good service is extremely unfair to your practice growth

Every act of goodness deserves to have no boundaries but just boundless reach. There are a number of people who need your service to better their lives.

So, you as a healthcare provider need to be telling people what difference you can bring in patients life because there is no patient going to shout from their rooftop that they are badly in need of help and are searching for a healthcare provider to seek help. While they are going to ask their near and dear ones if they knew a healthcare provider who is an expert in solving issues that they are suffering from. You reaching them at the right time through information is the best primary help you can do to your patients. Keeping your capabilities to yourself will defeat the very purpose of helping those in need.

5. Your result impacts your referral partner's reputation

Make sure the referrer also knows the exact patient journey of the case they are referring to. So that they feel confident about their suggestion of a healthcare brand and feel satisfied that they have actually helped somebody in need. If your referrer is personally very close to the referral make sure they are present with the patient at the peaks of a patient journey like the first initial consultation and other crucial stages to impart mutual confidence in the doctor-referrer relationship.

The promise that you deliver will add value to your referrer, they want to know how well you have served the referral they have given you so that their image and regard gets brownie points from the referral.

6 Consistency is growth

The moment you kick-start a referral program your duty is not over. Keeping your network functional and not static is the best way to go forward with your Word-of-Mouth marketing program.

Make sure to revive the funnel as periodic as possible to see the best results in your program, throughout the year plan activities from minute to big to help your Word-of-Mouth marketing program. Be it involving yourself in fraternity friendly events that have exclusive networking sessions, or attending CMEs- be consistent at it.

Follow up with the contact base you have developed for your own brand and make sure you segregate them according to their response. Keep filtering your funnel regularly so that the rate of your marketing effort efficiency increases to impact more people over time. Consistency in maintaining the strength of your referral marketing program decides how long it will work for you

7 Push your competitive edge forward

Your competitive edge is taking a step forward every day by trying to do new things every other day, as you try to do new things every day to improve your healthcare brand's effectiveness, that makes yours a dynamic brand. Crack a referral marketing program that adapts with your growth strategies as you look to grow.

Having a strong referral marketing program means that you will have a strong competitive edge amongst the others in your fraternity. Through this, you will know more doyens and, the more they know you they'll collaborate with you.

8 Evaluate your Word-of-Mouth marketing program

Track your referral program as to how it has been contributing to your Healthcare brand's growth. Periodically evaluate which referral partner of yours has been contributing more. Classify partners accordingly. Classify your group into hot, warm and lukewarm and work on it accordingly.

Referrers under the hot category are those who refer your patients, regularly. Understand the pattern of referrals and interact with them frequently to understand the scope for improvisation. Referrers under the warm category are those who refer you, patients in-frequently so spend time with them to understand their understanding about your brand and capabilities and share case studies that will be relevant to them. Referrers under the lukewarm category are those who are yet to build trust with the brand or they already have partners to whom they are referring. So, share constant communication which can build trust with referrers under this category.

9 Expand your network

There is no end to word-of-mouth marketing. Continuously add referral partners to align with your vision and mission. Keep increasing your referral partners to push your horizon forward.
Expand your referral network not blindly but in a targeted way. Targeted strategies can accelerate your healthcare brand's prospect acquisition in a lesser period of time allowing you to venture into more impactful areas through market expansion. This happens when you understand that all the referrers for your healthcare brand aren't alike and are trying to serve differently through their own unique network.

A referrer who knows more patients through their own practice of general medicine may refer you to a case you are expert in solving, whereas a specialist in the same area may call you only in case of acute complexity which you can handle well. So, understanding diversity and catering to it through your referral marketing strategy is better than shooting at all without an aim.

Go as per the nature of your referrer's practice and try to frame a strategy by grouping them. This indeed will be more effective for your healthcare brand's market growth in a short period of time.

Do you realize how much you have grown through this marketing technique without even having invested seriously in it? Word-of-Mouth Referral network actually decides your net worth as it always had, so it is high time that you see which part of the whole loaf you have been taking for granted all along. Take it seriously and invest little more effort and time to make your referral marketing program the base of building your healthcare brand. The best way to amplify the reach of your word-of-mouth marketing is by documenting their voice in the form of testimonies that can reach those in need and give them the confidence to opt for the brand services. The testimony has to be obtained with permission from the word of mouth agent.

Word-of-Mouth referral marketing is not a stand-alone strategy having one purpose of increasing the in-flow of patients alone but, soon you will start to realize that Word-of-Mouth referral marketing will compliment everything you are trying to achieve as a healthcare brand. Crack this secret formula of all successful brands and unleash the fullest potential of your healthcare brand.

4
WORD OF MOUTH
ACTION PLAN

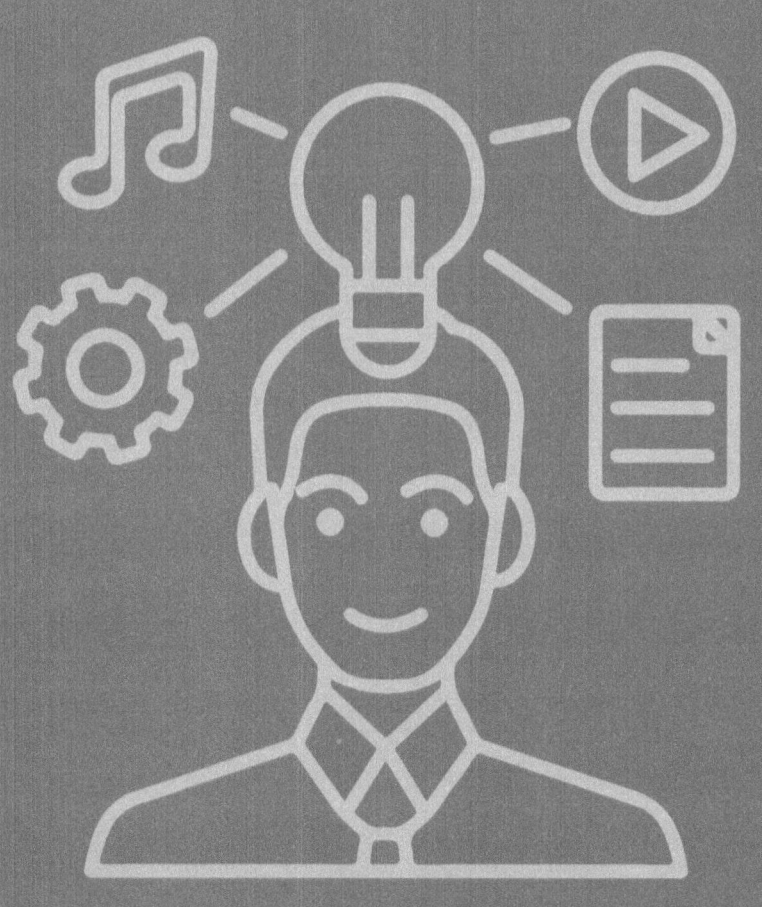

6 DEFECTS IN ORGANIC WORD-OF-MOUTH REACH WHICH WEAKENS ITS PERFORMANCE

01 BIASED & SUBJECTIVE
The person who delivers the information can be biased and subjective and may not deliver that information which is essentially to be delivered

02 INSUFFICIENT INFORMATION
The word-of-mouth agent may always not have enough information about the brand he is referring

03 CAN'T BE VERIFIED IN DEPTH
The word-of-mouth agent may actually not be a brand beneficiary, he might have learned about it from somewhere he/she does not remember where exactly.

04 PERSONAL INTEGRITY MATTERS
Brand Integrity depends on integrity of the word-of-mouth agent. If the word-of-mouth agent has less trust value, the brand he advocates also loses trust.

05 IS SLOW
Word-of-mouth reach is very slow. It depends on various factors like memory, right time, right place, right person, right need, right mood..etc.

06 BAD REPUTATION IS ALSO POSSIBLE
Brand adversaries can also propagate information about a brand which may not be true and people may not have the right means to verify the information.

3 STEP PLAN TO CREATE STRUCTURED ORGANIC WORD OF MOUTH REACH

1 STEP

GIVE THEM TOOLS

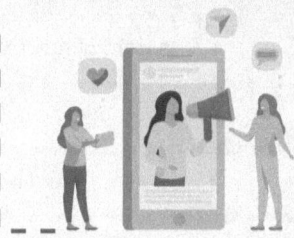

Keep Primary Audience Informed

Always make the primary audience more informed about your past & present legacy with constant communication. Use your hospital internal branding as an essential ingredient to communicate your legacy - people will pick up this message and amplify. When they are in your hospital they have every reason to learn more about you so make best use of this time to educate your primary audience

2 STEP

ANSWER WHEN THEY ASK

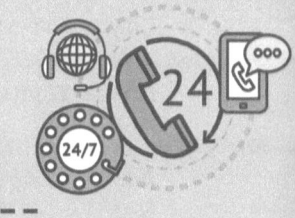

Build Brand Direct Communication Platforms

When people have any query about your brand who may be primary, secondary, tertiary agents or referred individuals, they should be able to directly verify about it with you - through your website / chat / call / whatsapp / direct visit, etc. Keep the brand direct communication open.

3 STEP

GIVE THEM THE PROOF TO PROVE THEY ARE RIGHT

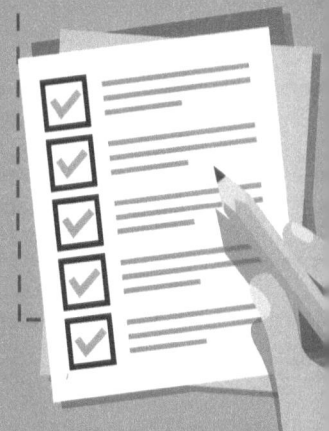

Make your Structured reach superior

Keep your brand audience informed about your current accomplishments via online and offline mediums which will make them feel proud about you, will rekindle memory about your brand and make the brand memory stronger, will trigger word-of-mouth about you on a consistent basis whenever the agent feels necessary, will bridge broken ties, will help them in upgrading your brand knowledge, when they talk about you they will talk about this latest happening first and you will make them win their conversation about you by giving proofs time and again. After a point it's not your brand it's their brand - they will be very personal about it, anyone hurting the brand will hurt their ego.

WORD OF MOUTH (WOM) MARKETING CHECKLIST

		Yes	No
1	Is word of mouth marketing working for you?	☐	☐
2	How do you evaluate the performance of your Word of Mouth?	☐	☐
3	Are your Word of Mouth agents increasing day-by-day?	☐	☐
4	Do you have any source to track your Word of Mouth agents?	☐	☐
5	Are you aware about the percentage of business contributed by Word of Mouth?	☐	☐
6	Do you have a medium to reach Word of Mouth agents?	☐	☐
7	Do your Word of Mouth agents understand your brand legacy well?	☐	☐
8	Are you taking initiative to update your Word of Mouth agents about the current happenings within the brand?	☐	☐
9	Are you inviting your Word of Mouth agents to participate in your various cause based initiatives?	☐	☐
10	Are your Word of Mouth agents getting in touch with you directly to verify/clarify any information about your brand?	☐	☐
11	Are you answering promptly when your Word of Mouth agents are asking any queries?	☐	☐
12	Do you have any feedback mechanism to evaluate your performance by your Word of Mouth agents?	☐	☐
13	Did you ever understand why some Word of Mouth agents have stopped referring you?	☐	☐
14	Do you understand why Word of Mouth agents want to refer your brand?	☐	☐
15	Do you do any Word of Mouth engagement exercise to keep them referring you?	☐	☐

STRATEGY 5

"THE MORE REAL IT IS, THE MORE RELIABLE IT GETS!"

PATIENT EXPERIENCE

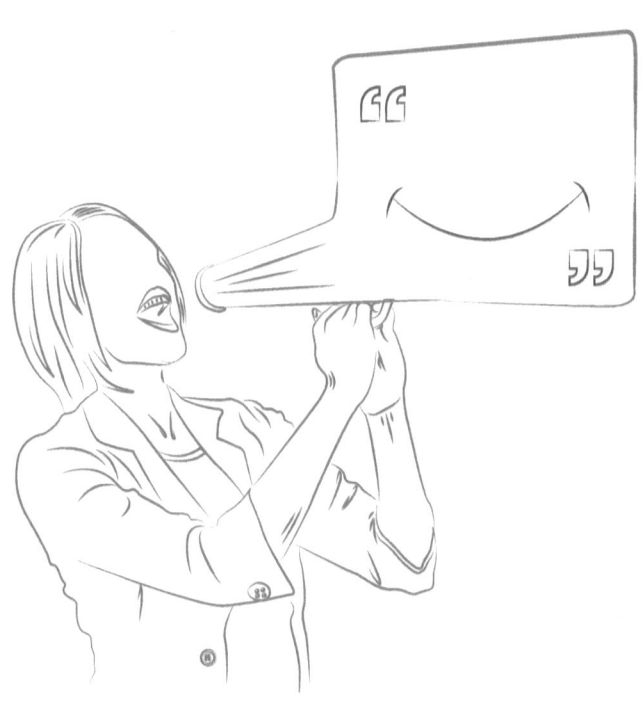

Experience Matters

Word of mouth marketing is the success formula for any brand promising its prospects a desirable experience. People advocate a brand based on the experience they have had with the brand, people when they feel happy and satisfied with your service they also feel the need to spread this good and let others also enjoy the experience that your brand promises. Patient experience marketing is all about getting that word of mouth marketing component more powerfully delivered through kindling the good at the right point and making that good reach the right doorsteps.

Since patient experiences are the anchoring factors to your word of mouth presence it is important that you keep the patient-centric approach in mind while planning each element in your hospital. You never know which element is making great patient experiences or breaking the same so make sure you have a system in place to get to know it. It is not just about creating quality content through documenting patient experiences but it also reveals your blind spots and lets you create a patient-friendly habitat that breeds seamless experience for each one inside your hospital. This indeed contributes to the betterment of your hospital in the true sense of what patients actually expect out of you.

When patient experiences are recorded in various ways and approaches, it can make good reach others who are in need of the same experience. Patient experiences are the verified, credible and most realistic answers you are giving your future prospects on why they should be choosing you and for what they should choose you for. Patient experience becomes that ultimate type of content that can escalate the effectiveness of your marketing outreach plan by accelerating brand visibility, desirability and reliability at once!

!!CAUTION!!
4 Don'ts with Patient Experience Marketing

1 Avoid forced testimonials

Patient Experiences are not to be obtained forcefully or published without consent; it is a voluntary act of patients who are looking to narrate their story so that they can share a ray of hope to those affected with similar difficulties or as a token of gratitude to the doctor or organization.

2 Avoid scripted testimonials

Avoid publishing synthesized or scripted emotional testimonials which will ruin your brand reputation as people are smart enough to understand. Also, it is found many hospitals add fake positive reviews to their Google My Business page which can easily be found, so avoid it.

3. Avoid doctor in the video

It is an unethical practice to have a video testimonial where the patient is accompanied by the doctor as the testimonial is narrated. It looks like the doctor is directly soliciting patients through this testimonial which is against the guidelines.

4. Avoid intentional/non-intentional harm to other brands

Patients in the run of explaining their positive experience with you may tend to intentionally/un-intentionally harm other brands. So, before publishing such experiences kindly ensure you duly edit them.

Patient experience contains four different parts to it:

I. Patient Experience Creation
II. Patient Experience Collection
III. Patient Experience Marketing
IV. Patient Experience Management

I. Patient Experience Creation

Good patient experiences are created through absolutely integrated process that puts patients first and has a patient centric approach in every given nuance and detail that could probably decide the nature of a patient's experience in a hospital. Once that is set right patients will start to experience effortlessly satisfactory service from your side, which makes them bless your brand. The blessing indeed is the word-of-mouth-marketing they generate, it creates a ripple effect when used for marketing your brand through reliably noble ways.

"Unless the experience itself is good, it cannot be marketed"

From suffering to cure, from hesitation to happiness travel with them, be involved in every moment of the patient journey

Every patient journey says more about your capabilities as a healthcare brand and practitioner more than the patient. Bring along a great amount of compassion at every step to win the trust of your patient. Count on those small details that could mean big to your patients, maybe their whole experience with your healthcare brand will be a summed up one based on those little things you offer to comfort your patient.

Aim to win trust at each step, at each step of the patient journey the doctor and the team that interacts and travels with the patient and the convenience factor all are key deciding parameters for the whole experience your healthcare brand stands for. At each step be equally concerned and efficient.

Every tinge of effort counts

Every healthcare brand invests its maximum efforts to keep the levels of their patient satisfaction high. Each initiative taken contributes to the ultimate result. But do people know that you have taken such initiatives. Your patients love to be told that you are adding as much value to their patient experience as it expected from you.

Create moment of truths

"Moment of Truth" is that moment with your brand a patient experiences first hand when you deliver on your promise. If the brand delivers then the patient understands the brand promise to be true to its promise and becomes an effective brand advocate. If the promise is not delivered, then it carries a bad brand experience.

Create as many "moments of truth" as possible which you have promised your potential patients to provide quality care and much more. When you promise your patients a seamless healthcare experience and deliver exactly the same, your credibility increases in manifolds and the end goal of attaining the highest level of patient satisfaction is achieved. At each touchpoint you make or break your impression so, take ardent care in delivering the promise.

Moments of Truth are unforgettable experiences in a patient's lifetime and will become an effective tool in the minds of the patients to guard the brand when they see someone spreading misinformation about the brand. The moment of truth they experienced gives them the confidence to speak for your brand. What they see through their own eyes and hear directly has far more impact than anything, that's the power of "Moments of Truth."

11. Patient Experience Collection

Patient experience collection can serve a lot more than just the aim of marketing your healthcare brand. Collecting patient experience multiplies the result and its soft impact in the heart of patients. Make your happy patients realize that their happiness should not just start and end. It should rather create hope of cure to millions who are suffering with similar ailments.

Let the experienced talk for the experience

The best way to market the patient experience your brand is set to give, is by making your past patients talk about the experience they received. Let them express their happiness and satisfaction in their own way, the quality of patient experience becomes more desirable when there is a great amount of gratitude and emotional quotient showered in it.

Be mindful about how and when to collect

Collecting patient testimonials and stories related to the healthcare experience can turn out to be a journey defining moment with your patient. There are really emotional points where the patients feel the peak of gratitude for the healthcare brand and the doctor which is also the right moment to approach for a testimonial as the feelings expressed will be more organic and straight from the heart.

Create the aura around for encouraging patients to share their experience, focus more on how people are getting benefitted through testimonials, patients will voluntarily come forward to share their review to make a difference to someone's life. This can happen through simple posters that say "Share your Story" or "Pass on Hope" to really keep the goodness going or messages in your social media and website will also help collect experiences by showcasing already recorded experiences and prompting them to share their story.

Collect patient testimonials in varied formats

Collecting patient testimonials in varied formats makes the end result of the whole plan more effective in terms of versatility. Only when testimonials are collected in different formats such as questionnaire, a written letter of gratitude for the doctor or a video mostly preferred of all the above it can reach as many as possible in the desired way. Also, have eye-catching interior branding posters in your hospital that attracts Google reviews so your online presence is strengthened.

III Patient Experience Marketing

Patient experience marketing is perhaps the best and most crucial step that serves the important purpose of telling the world what big difference your healthcare brand has created in people's lives. Give your healthcare brand the right kind of marketing input it deserves through authentic and really reliable content like patient experience anecdotes to find the best results.

Different formats for different impacts

Patient experience can be collected in different channels for marketing in different ways for a wide range of reach and visibility for the brand. With so many varied mediums and channels, patient experience can be marketed effectively.

Narrate it to the right ones, at the right time

Reach the stories of happy patient experience through the right mediums to the right audiences. Making sure that these stories that reach your potential patients are the effective ways of spreading your horizon and letting your brand make a real-time appeal to people who may actually need your services.

Where is more important than how

Placing the marketing communication created through patient experience is an act that can determine the effectiveness of your patient experience marketing plan. The communication created through this can be used for interior branding, online content marketing, media publications and etc.

Create a ripple effect in the sea of goodness

Have a holistic goal for your whole marketing plan, realize the impact potential of patient experience marketing. The very act of passing on a patient experience anecdote can mean an act of goodness in itself. When a satisfied patient accounts for their experience and vouches for the healthcare brand, they develop so much hope in people who need healthcare solutions. When a patient experience reaches a million other patients it creates a better impact which not only benefits the hospital but the entire set of people who need the confidence to overcome their illness/ailments.

IV. Patient Experience Management

Patient Experience Management is about aligning the outcome of each patient experience with the ultimate goal of helping more patients through reliable stories continuously. There are certain precautions you need to take before taking a plunge into patient experience marketing. Make your plan and its goals stay well within the rules to really make it big through patient experience marketing and not have a second thought about it.

Handle with care

Details revealed to market patient experience has to be genuine Maintain the utmost sensitivity to pain points and narrate them without sounding too hard proving your capabilities. Your brand perception should be a result of pure trust, not gullibility.

Realize that being loud does not make you the most heard!

There is absolutely no second thought about the importance of narrating patient stories but the way you narrate them is more important. Be conscious & make sure the lines of persuasion don't merge with exaggeration that could probably hinder the loyalty that your brand has already earned.

Good ones don't express so the not so good ones naturally stand out

People consider it as normal to receive good treatment and care from their healthcare brands, as a healthcare brand looking to market your patient experience take necessary steps to kindle the good and bring out happy patient experiences. So encourage them to share their story.

Keep up the act of spreading good

Create systems in place and educate your staff on the importance of creating positive patient experiences, make necessary changes wherever required to create beautiful experiences. Reward the partners and the staff who upkeep the patient experiences. By creating a well-informed team, which has patient experience as the core priority which inturn infuses this mantra into the brand culture is destined to be far ahead of others.

Patient Experience Marketing is perhaps the noblest way of making stories of satisfaction multiply further through effectively passing on the message. Anything that you are doing to increase the quality of service and better any aspect of your healthcare brand ultimately boils down to the patient experience. So, make sure you create the best experiences for your patients and then, tell the world that you are set out to create the best healthcare experiences.

The key to increasing the efficiency of your healthcare brand is in making happy patient stories reach the right people at the right time. This indeed will rejuvenate ray of hopes, reduce the fear of ailment and move people from viewing sickness as stoppage blocks in their life. Patient experience marketing is all about spreading good results and making people believe in the cure and power of healing. Support the power of a patient's voice

Note

5
PATIENT EXPERIENCE
ACTION PLAN

STEPS INVOLVED IN
PATIENT EXPERIENCE CAPTURE

TALK TO THEM

After a successful treatment, if patients express their gratitude. You can suggest them if they prefer they can share a testimonial which can help others like them

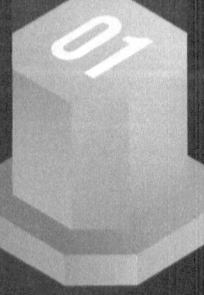 01

FREEZE THE TYPE

If they are interested, then you can collect testimonial as per patient convenience in the form of written text in email, Google Review, Video & Audio.

02

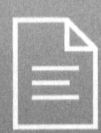

DOCUMENT IT

Have a clear documentation of all your testimonies in various forms in sufficient back ups, they are real treasure and ageless

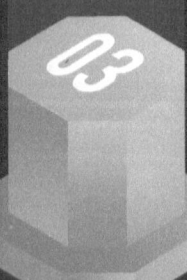 03

PUBLISH IT

Publish them in your case studies, quote as references in your research and use them in your online mediums

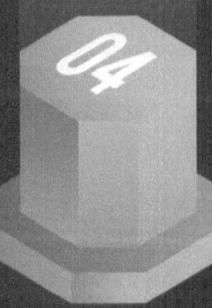 04

3 TYPES OF PATIENT EXPERIENCE CAPTURE VIA VIDEOS

1. PATIENT STORY FORM
Where story is narrated by the patient, their journey from pain and suffering to healthy and normal life.

2. CASE STUDY FORM
Wherein the script has to cover the story from doctor and the patient. Doctor can use medical terminologies as it will be presented to mixed audience from fraternity and general public. It has to be more educative in nature.

3. MOTIVATION MESSAGE FORM
This type gives confidence to the those affected by same disease wherein a recovered patients gives hope saying 'I have recovered and you too can'

CHECKLIST
FOR PATIENT TESTIMONIAL

		Yes	No
1	Do you showcase your testimonies in your waiting area?	☐	☐
2	Do you have a poster in your waiting area which encourages people to share testimonies ?	☐	☐
3	Do you showcase the positive impact which is created by your patient testimonies which have helped others?	☐	☐
4	Do you use your patient testimonies in your marketing efforts?	☐	☐
5	Have you obtained permissions for all your testimonies from your respective patients in written format for their use online / offline?	☐	☐
6	Do you take learnings from your testimonials and implement them for smooth patient journey?	☐	☐
7	Do you showcase these testimonies to your staff to motivate on the positive direction the brand is heading?	☐	☐
8	Did you create a BOOK of TESTIMONIALS and keep it at your patient waiting area?	☐	☐

FIND ANSWERS FOR THESE, IT WILL HELP

Which medium people prefer to give testimonies to you?

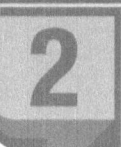
When you ask them for testimonies what difficulties you face?

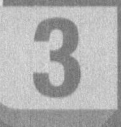
What are the elements you use in your touch points which can encourage people to give positive testimonies?

Note

STRATEGY 6

"THE DIGITAL FUTURE IS NOW. PLAY IT AS IT EVOLVES!"

DIGITAL MARKETING

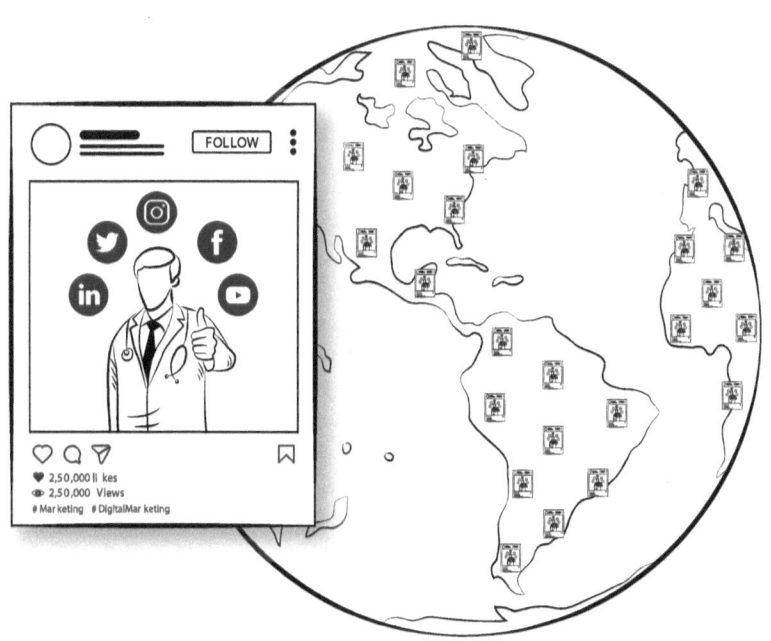

The Digital Game Begins now

Digital Marketing is the new now, it is the way to reach your prospects. Digital Marketing is the way people are making decisions today, no matter how near or far you are, your digital presence is a big influencing factor for your patients to make a healthcare decision. People look for healthcare providers, health information and everything that is health online to arrive at the right decision, if you are a practitioner from the traditional school then digital marketing is sure to take you by surprise.

But don't get baffled, all that digital marketing requires from your side, is initiative and efforts. Take the right steps and have a dedicated plan or strategy throughout your digital marketing journey. Don't do it because the medium and the millennial generation demand it, but do it because your brand asks for it from within. When the purpose is well defined, you can act on it and do what exactly is expected out of your brand from your prospects.

7 Commandments of Digital Marketing Strategy

1 You were just searched! Were you found?

Patients are now searching for their doctors online. Nearly all of them go to doctor shopping online when they need to find a new doctor or the doctor they get to know through their network. A strong web presence will help them find you easily.

Even if you practice the next door of your patient, he/she is going to search for you online. Their decision will fully depend on your online presence and how strong you have established it to be. The main motivating factor for people to make decisions on their healthcare practitioners is online reputation.

When people find you, what do they look for?
They want the brand to be original, transparent & communicative.

Stay Original - Stay who you are, irrespective of what new marketing strategy you are looking to venture into. The key to being sustainably successful at digital marketing is to stay yourself and capitalize on that originality factor. People will love you for who you are, if your online personality and offline personality don't clash, but complement each other.

Stay Transparent - Transparency in showing what your digital audience wants to see in your practice or your hospital is more important. Your brand will also stand out by frequency of audience engagement as the content's reliability quotient is high.

Stay Communicative - The audience wants the communication to be two way. Especially when it comes to health-related issues it is better to hear people out to keep them satisfied which will also fulfills your duty as a healthcare provider.

2. Be omnipresent

Your potential patients and current patients can access information everywhere. People don't select and choose platforms when they want to consume information. Making use of every platform to its own benefit is what digital marketing calls for.

Choose several mediums that need content that you are looking to create. Understand that content of your medical expertise is required in different forms by different mediums that let users engage differently and act accordingly.

3. Your people read, remember, recall, reach, review and refer. Cash the gold at every point!

It's not just about being up and alive in all digital platforms but it is about making oneself matter to the target audience by etching your personality through web presence.

How you stay relevant to today's audience is the key to opening. Have a unified strategy to make the biggest impact on your patient's daily feed. People are taking your online image as seriously as your offline so at every point make a mark.

4. Educate before you promote

Always remember that there are people who may not need you at the moment to solve their health issue but are however interested in getting a health information download. So educate through your professional expertise and knowledge about your specialty. Be that authentic source of information people are searching for.

5. The content bank is the digital treasure

Content is the king. The majority agree to have searched something about health almost every day on Google. Content, not just about doctor and hospital, but on general health education is always looked out for by your potential patients. Serve the need!

6. Make your content Personal & Relevant

A content that speaks to the world reaches none, but a content that speaks to one reaches the world. Make your content touch each one of your potential patients. Analyze needs and wants through interaction and create content catering the same.

7. Establish a strong communication

Stand up and talk for yourself, facilitate direct communication for your brand through authentic channels to increase the authenticity quotient in the information. Keep your merit guarded through strong web presence, let no similar ones take the credit for your achievement.

Digital Game is evolving every day and more serious decisions are made online. This platform demands a good amount of attention which is generally ignored, as much importance is given to offline platforms for promotion, so is the importance needed to be given for online platforms. A perfect mix of online backed by offline is the need of the hour.

6

DIGITAL MARKETING
ACTIVITY

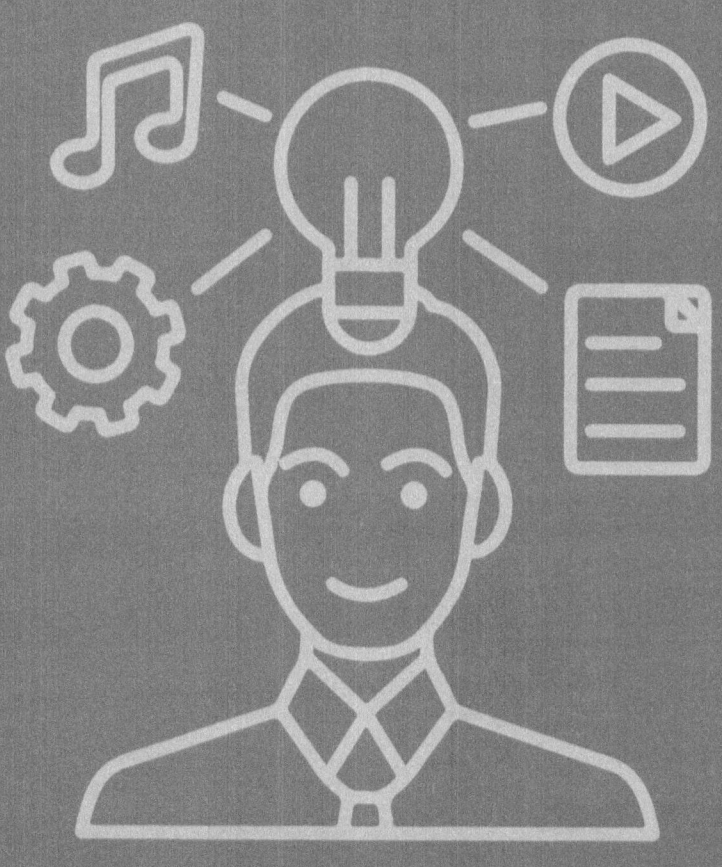

5 Search Method
Find your patients as your patients find you

5 Search Method is for all those who have little or no knowledge in digital marketing. By simply following these search methods you can serve your patients.

5 Search Method is formulated after thoroughly understanding how patients find information about a hospital brand online. We have encountered 5 important search journeys patients undertake to find their healthcare partner. Each journey reveals a unique story behind the search. It is only wise to be competent in all the search areas to create a satisfying experience.

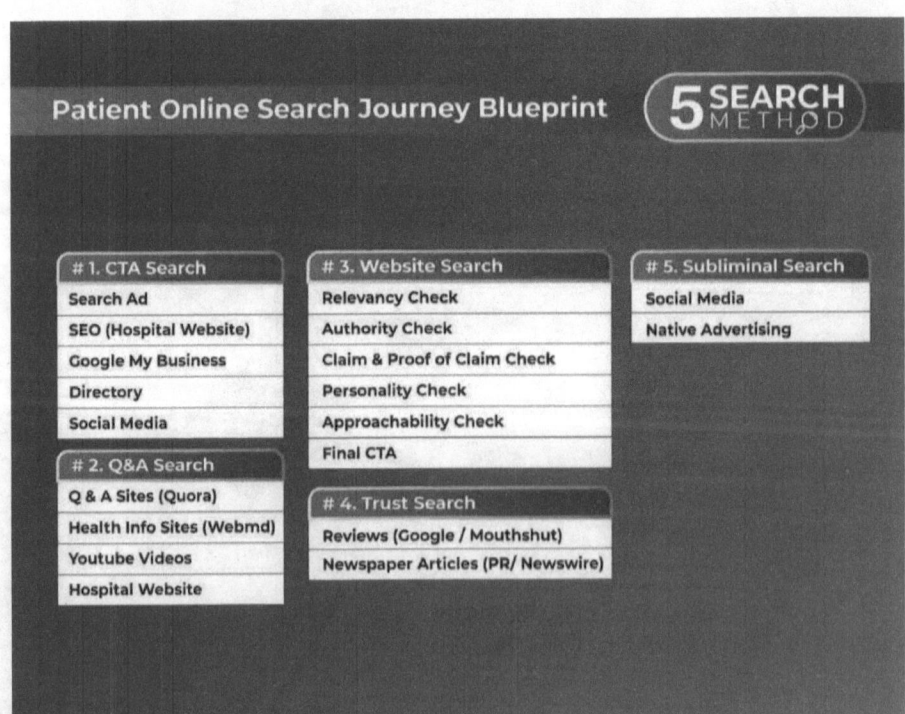

Why it is Important to Consider implementing the essentials in 5 Search Method

1. Answer before they ask: Each search method is a solution to the question people are asking in their journey.

2. Be there before they find you: Being there before they find you is the easiest way to find you when they want to reach you to fix up an appointment or need more info.

3. No Hassle Approach: You dont have to understand the complexity of digital marketing. If you understand how patients approach you, you can work accordingly.

4. No Sequence Approach: Patients may pick up any search method in their journey. So make your search results in all 5 approaches sound.

5. No Confusion Approach: By simply following this and improvising your performance based on these search methods, you can be assured of fabulous results.

Search Method #1
Call-To-Action (CTA) Search

> Are you easy to find when Im searching you Online?

When people decide to find your contact details online to fix up an appointment, are you easily approachable?. If there is difficulty in people contacting you despite being interested to contact you, that's is the biggest trouble you are creating to your brand audience. It's also injustice to your brand searchers online.

This search method is frequently adopted by patients/prospects who are aware of your hospital brand or are particular about finding a specialist, but dont have your contact details tocontact you. So, they search online to find your contact information. They are the hot prospects who need your immediate attention more than anybody else.

Hot prospects need immediate contact information to connect with you. If you miss to catch them here you lose them.

There are 5 types of results your prospects may encounter when they are doing CTA Search.

Patient Online Search Journey Blueprint

5 SEARCH METHOD

1. CTA Search
Search Ad
SEO (Hospital Website)
Google My Business
Directory
Social Media

Search Ad

The first search result people get is that of google adwords. Never miss the opportunity to rank first.

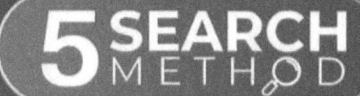

Ad · www.chennaifertilitycenter.com/ ▼ 096411 65197
Best Fertility Clinic Chennai | High Success Rate
Advanced **Fertility** Treatment **Clinic in Chennai** with Expert Doctors. 23,000+ Success Babies. High Success Rate. We Help You Make Your Baby Dreams Come True. Request An Appointment Now. Experienced Technicians. One Stop **Center**.
📍 79/129, Nelson Manickam Road, Opp Raymond Showroom, Aminjikarai, Chennai, Tamil Nadu

Ad · www.novaivffertility.com/ ▼
Nova IVF Center In Chennai | Guidance From Counsellors Team
Continuous Guidance From a Supportive Team Of Counsellors. Ask A **Fertility** Specialist. Bringing Happiness To Childless Couples.Ethical Treatments & Transparent Pricing.

SEO
This helps your website rank in the first page of google in the organic listing. You can pick a few keywords based on analytics and rank for them

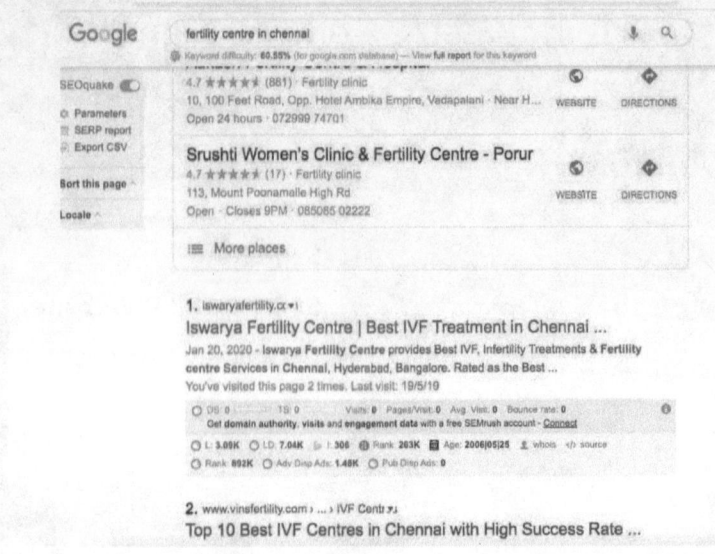

Google My Business
This is the smartest tool developed by Google. It shows directions to your business location, records reviews, working hours, contact information and more. Getting listed here will give you unique advantage when you are geographically closer to your prospect.

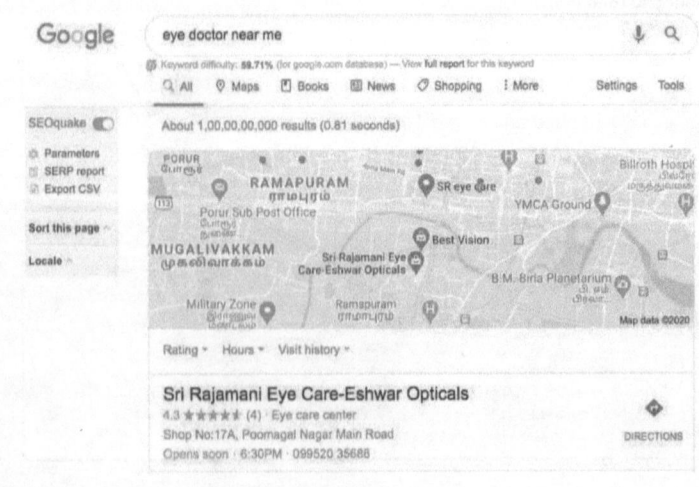

Directory

Getting your organisation details in local directories is good. These local directories are very popular with your prospects and powerful in SEO, may connect you to your relevant audience.

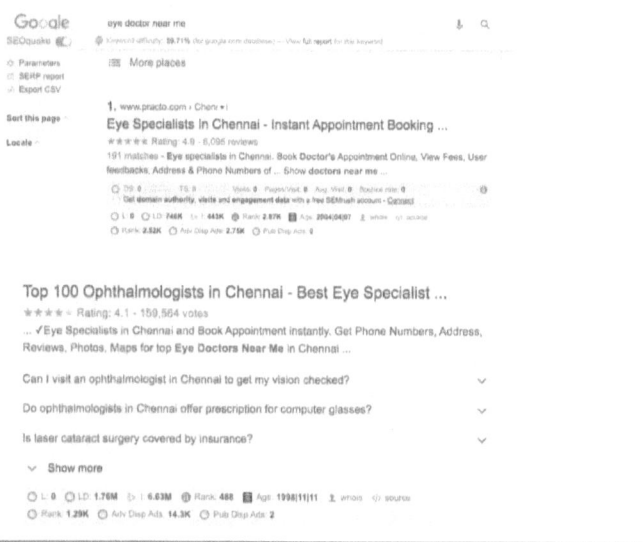

Social Media

Sometimes in the brand search results your social media handles may pop-up make sure your contact information is updated there as well.

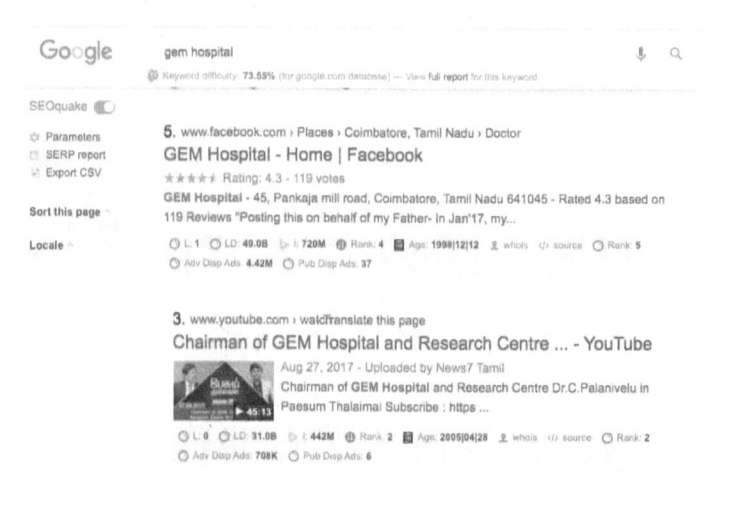

Search Method #2
Question & Answer (Q&A) Search

> Are you willing to help me?

Under this search method, you prospect undertakes the journey of finding answer for health related questions. They may have some complications or their dear ones may have some complications, when they hear those terms from their doctor - they started googling to find more about that complication and resultant treatment for cure.

When your brand can help the prospect in clarifying the health doubts by answering their FAQs in your website or in sites like Quora, you stand to gain their attention. Through education you build trust and then they would be interested to find more about your services and opt.

Quality Content is the key. So make sure the content is accurate, highly informative and presented in simple terms with less medical jargons.

People when they search with a question they may get search results from the following and are likely to get educated through these sources.

Patient Online Search Journey Blueprint

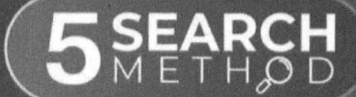

 # 2. Q&A Search

| Q & A Sites (Quora) |
| Health Info Sites (Webmd) |
| Youtube Videos |
| Hospital Website |

Q & A Sites

Sites like Quora where people ask a lot of questions tops the list. Try answering their queries pertaining to your specialty in quota - you will not only answer them but also many others who are looking for the answers to the same question using quora.

dental implants cost in chennai

Keyword difficulty: **62.40%** (for google.com database) — View full report for this keyword
Rank: **1.69M**   Adv Disp Ads: **0**   Pub Disp Ads: **0**

3. www.quora.com › How-much-do-dental-implants-cost-in-Chennai
How much do dental implants cost in Chennai? - Quora
7 answers
Oct 12, 2017 - Good quality **implants** starts from Rs.20000 in **Chennai**.
Which is the best **cost**-effective hospital for a **dental** ...   5 answers   10 Apr 2018

Health Info Sites

Sites like WebMD that contain huge repository of health related information easily come top on the search results. If not in WebMD but in sites that carry such repository you can add your articles based on your specialty to answer the audience.

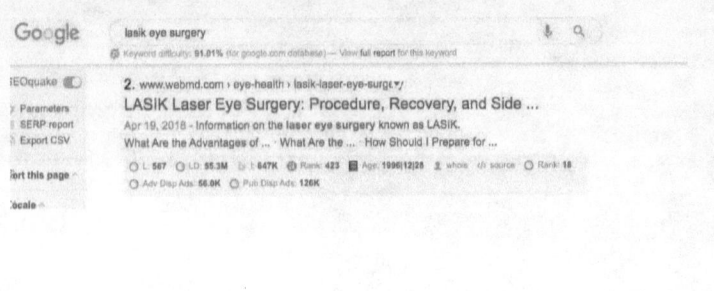

Youtube Videos

People nowadays search youtube to find answers for health related information, as the information comes in 3d visuals or actual video, people get to clarify their doubts easily. So create videos answering for the frequently asked questions and upload in youtube to reach wider audience. Make the video in English and Regional language.

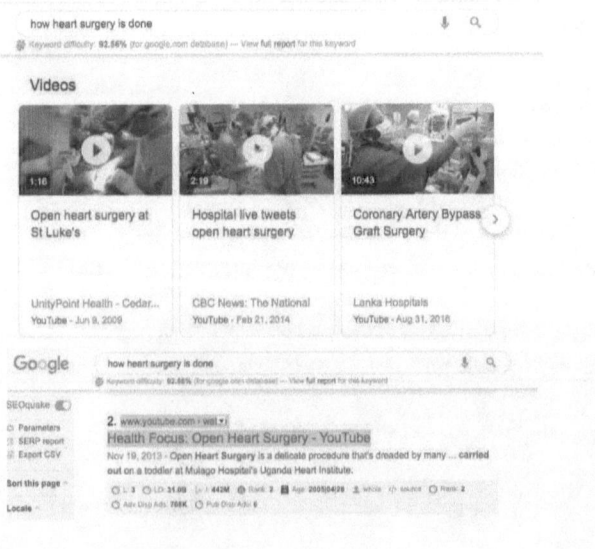

Hospital Website

Make sure for each specialty / treatment your hospital website has dedicated FAQs section where the frequently asked questions are mentioned and then relevant answers are provided in text, visuals and video content.

---

dental implants cost in chennai

Keyword difficulty: **62.40%** (for google.com database) — View **full report** for this keyword

Q All □ Images ⊘ Shopping ▶ Videos 📰 News ⋮ More   Settings Tools

About 4,57,000 results (0.49 seconds)

Ad · www.rajandental.com/dental/clinic ▼ 073389 65659

Dental Implants India | Compare Prices & Read Reviews

Affordable **Dental** Treatment in India - Book Today! 60 years experience; World class **dental implant** centre; Online consultation; American/UK Certified **dentists**; Lifetime Warranty. MALO CLINIC Collaboration. Services: Rootcanal Treatment, All-on-4 Treatment, Sedation **Dentistry**. Dental Implants · Zygoma Implant · All On 4 Implants · Get in Touch

Typically, a single **dental implant cost in Chennai** ranges between INR 18,000-45,000. This is only the **dental implant cost** and the **tooth** crown or denture **cost** is usually additional.

www.drsmilez.com › Services
Dental Implant cost in Chennai, India | Best Dental Implant ...

About Featured Snippets   Feedback

Search Method #3
Website Search

Are you convincing enough?

When patients/ prospects look at your website, they look at certain essentials which can build trust instantly with your brand. They have reached your website either by clicking your ad trying to learn more about your brand or heard about your brand through your word-of-mouth agent. Now, is your turn to give them the evidence they can trust instantly.

In lesser clicks if people can find the information they want, then thats the website which can fulfil the purpose. They may visit to check who you are, the management, specialties, doctor profiles, your merits & milestones and contact information.

When people go through your website, they check for the following to build trust.

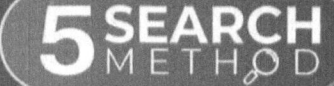

Relevancy Check

People first want to understand if they have landed in the official brand website which is offering treatments in that particular specialty they heard of

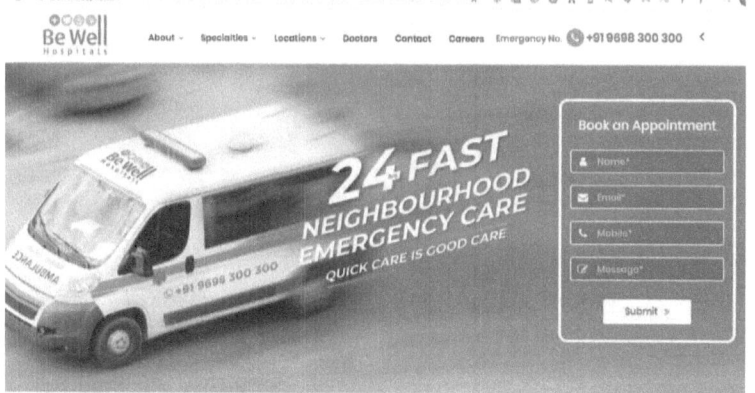

Authority Check

How confident is the brand in providing that particular treatment in the speaciality How the brand is regarded in the Industry. The face of the brand, numbers and case studies play a major role here

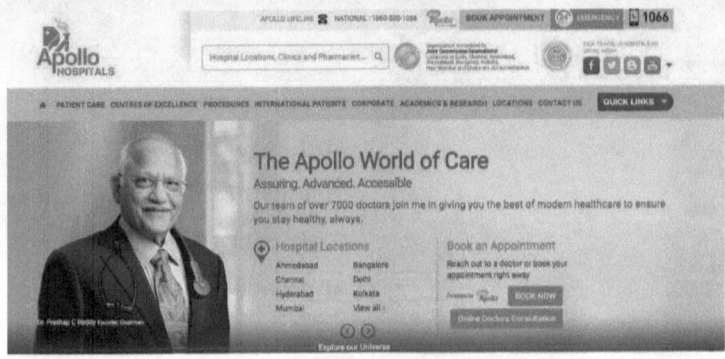

Claim and Proof of claim

When a brand claims to be a leader in a specific speciality, the proofof that claim will be checked. Testimonials count here.

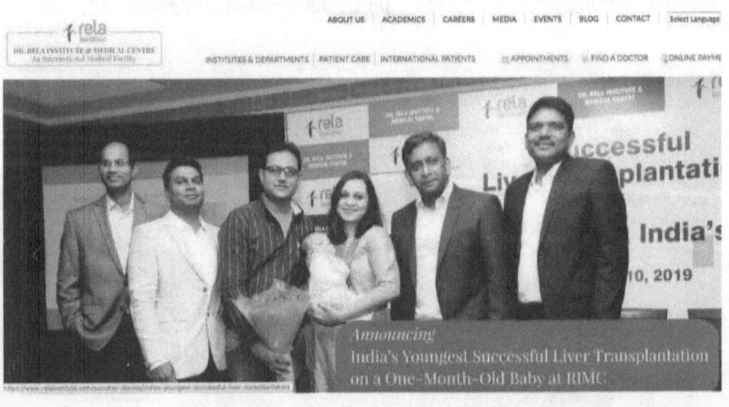

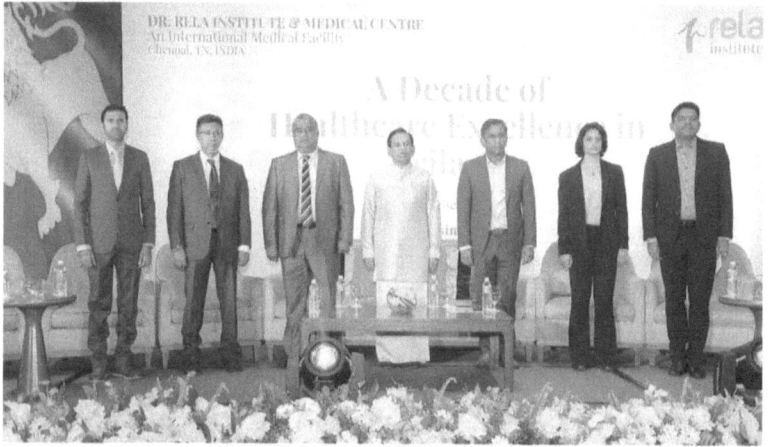

RIMC – Celebrates 10 years of Clinical Excellence with Sri Lankan patients

Personality Check

What is the tone of communication, that the brand is using in the website to narrate the brand story. People will want to know if it is a humble, sincere, transparent management?

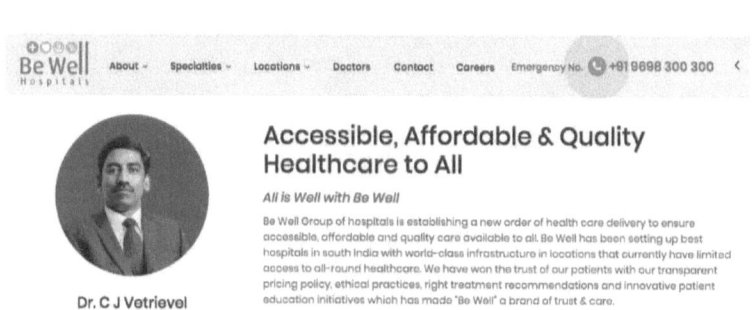

Approachability Check

People will want to reach the brand in various different ways and will want to know if the brand is easily reachable through multiple mediums, whether it be Chatbots, Enquiry forms, Emails, Cloud telephony and Social Media Messengers

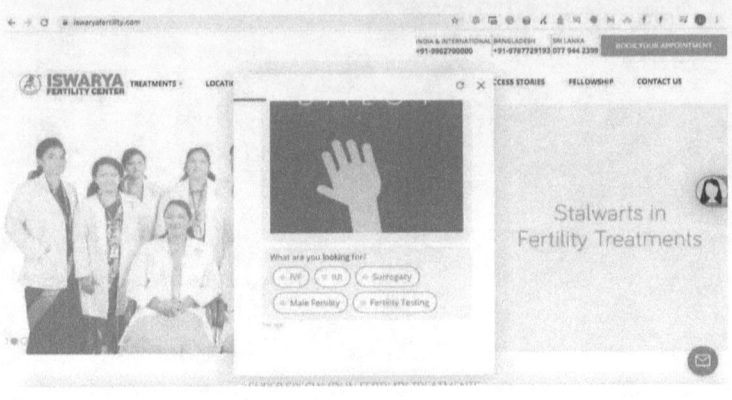

Final CTA

When they are convinced highlight either booking form or contact number as the strong thread to connect with the brand. Make these two or one prominent.

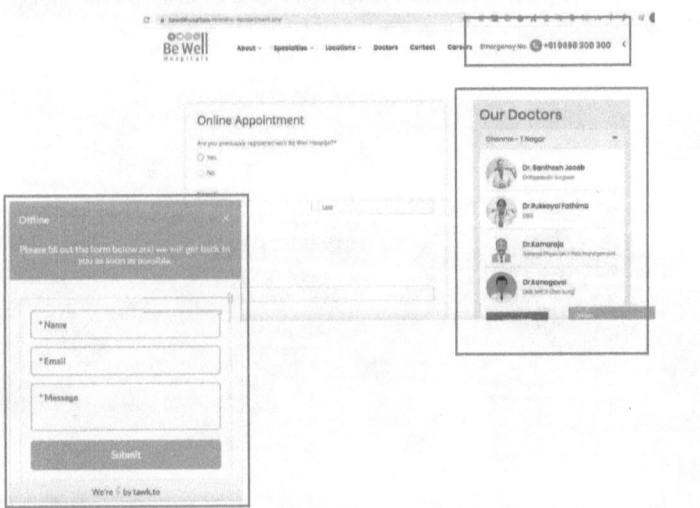

Search Method # 4
Trust Search

Are you Trustworthy?

This search method is used when the prospect has made up his / her mind to opt the brand but is still doubtful and wants some social proof from outside brand sources for final CTA.

In this method, the prospect checks google reviews and sites like mouthshut to understand if the brand has any positive or negative reviews and if so what are those. Based on this, he / she develops a brand reputation in the mind which can build or break trust with the brand.

It's advisable to keep constant check with the help of google alerts to understand if there are any brand mentions in the google to immediately act.

People check outside sources to build trust and they are as follow.

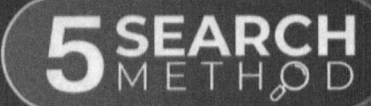

Review Sites

Review tools like Google My Business and sites like Mouthshut play a vital role in forming a positive brand image. Make sure you

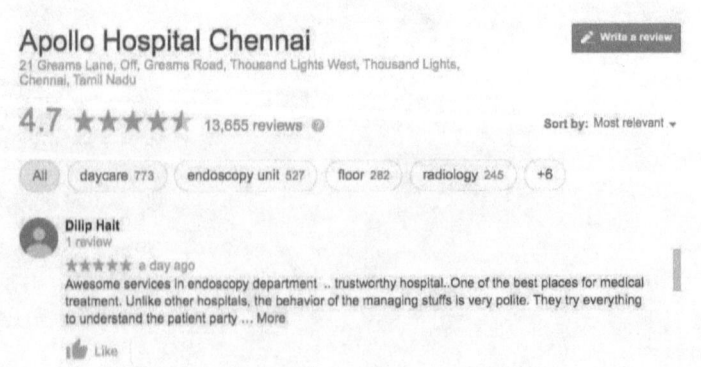

Press Release

You can do press release on major milestones. This will build up your image. You can also write articles on varied health subjects relating to your specialty which can appear in leading news papers.

Google — apollo hospital

All   Maps   News   Images   Shopping   More   Settings   Tools

About 2,07,000 results (0.36 seconds)

Apollo Hospitals Hosts Walkathon to Create Awareness About ...
Business Wire India (press release) - 3 hours ago
Right to Left: Mr. Santosh Marathe, Unit Head and COO, **Apollo Hospitals**, Navi Mumbai, Dr. Tejinder Singh, Consultant, Medical Oncologist, ...

Odisha: Cadaveric Transplant Patient Discharged From **Apollo** ...
Ommcom News - 10-Feb-2020
Bhubaneswar: The Doctors of Transplant Institute of **Apollo Hospitals**, Bhubaneswar gave a new life to a critically sick patient, Ghanashyam ...
Naveen felicitates SCB, **Apollo** Doctors For Odisha's 1st ...
Pragativadi - 22 hours ago
View all

CM Naveen Patnaik assures to provide help for organ ...
The New Indian Express - 11 hours ago
The doctors of transplant institute of **Apollo Hospitals**, Bhubaneswar, have given new life to Ghanashyam Jena.
CM Naveen Patnaik Congratulates SCB and **Apollo** Doctors ...
Kalinga TV - 10 hours ago
View all

Search Method # 5
Subliminal Search

> **Are you creating interest in me?**

People, most of the times do not (don't) say what they want, but subliminally are searching for answers to varied problems that they may have. In such cases subliminal search plays a dominant role.

In this type of search, the prospect is actually not searching but googling or visiting their social media sites to consume the content they want - in such a scenario they discover our content which they may be actually looking for which can be in the form of Facebook / Insta ads or through native advertising.

Lets understand these two types.

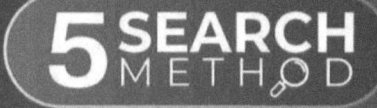

Social Media Ads

Based on the demographic and interest data and with social media platforms like Facebook or Instagram, we can precisely target people who are likely to be interested in your offerings.

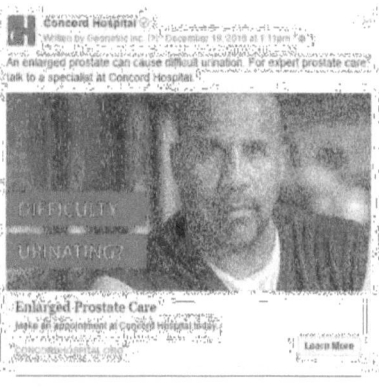
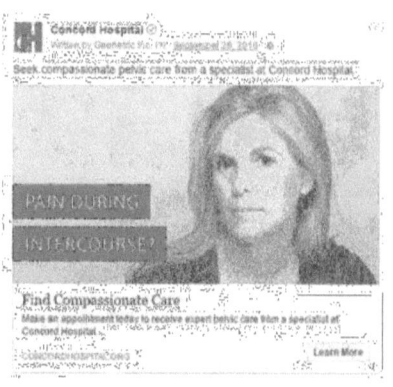

Native Advertising

This form of content placement is increasing and is used by brands of all genres of all genre and it is interesting to find many top hospital brands using it. Platforms like Taboola will place your content in popular news sites which can generate massive traffic. This method particularly will work when you have some wonder case studies or new technology - some curiosity creating factor or rare factor is necessary to pull the readers to read your content.

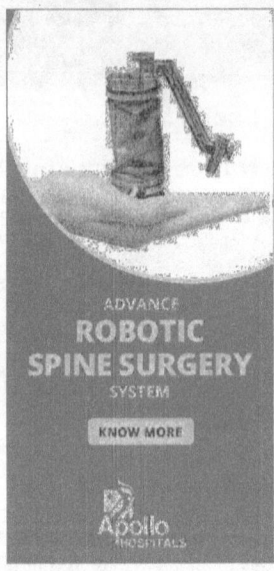
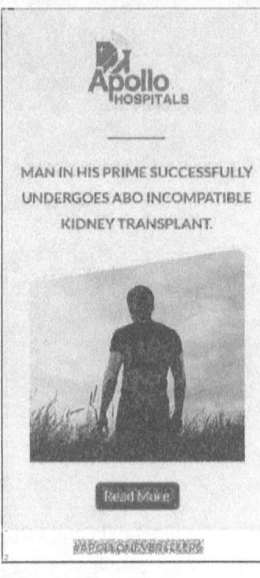
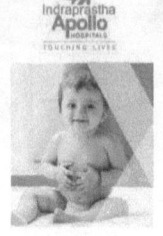

Behindwoods as a platform

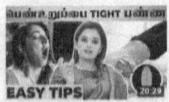

"50% Women Mas**bate பன்றாங்க" - Dr.Deepa Ganesh Explains | Cosmetic Gynecologist
SouthScope Tamil · 307K views · 2 months ago · 98%
"50% Women Mas**bate பன்றாங்க" - Dr.Deepa Ganesh Explains | Cosmetic Gynecologist OG Laser & Cosmetic...

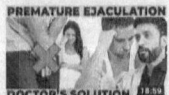

இப்படி Masturbation செய்தால் பீரச்சனை வராது - Doctor Karthick Gunasekaran விளக்கம்
Behindwoods Air · 437K views · 4 months ago · 95%
Subscribe - https://goo.gl/oMHseY We will work harder to generate better content. Thank you for your support. Reach 7 crore ...

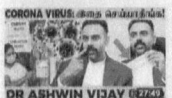

Corona Virus வந்திதிகள்.. யாரும் பயப்படாதீங்க - Dr Ashwin Vijay விளக்கம்
Behindwoods Air · 122K views · 1 week ago ·
Subscribe - https://goo.gl/oMHseY We will work harder to generate better content. Thank you for your support. Reach 7 crore ...

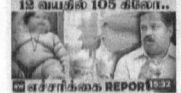

நோய் இல்லாமல் ஆரோக்கியமா வாழ இதை செய்யுங்க - Doctor Sivaraman interview
Behindwoods Air · 12K views · 1 month ago · 98%
Subscribe - https://goo.gl/oMHseY We will work harder to generate better content. Thank you for your support. Reach 7 crore ...

HOSPITAL WEBSITE CHECKLIST

 Call-to-Action

- Phone Number
- Appointment Form
- Address
- Google My Business Direction
- Consultation Timing
- Chat / Whatsapp

 **Essentials**

- Services / Treatments Offered
- Infrastructure
- Doctors & Their Profile
- About your Fertility Centre
- Insurance Details

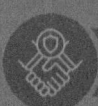 **Trust Builders**

- Video Testimonies of Patients
- Milestones
- Google Reviews (If your review are good)
- Awards / Accolades
- Case Studies
- Media /PR Snippets

HOSPITAL WEBSITE CHECKLIST

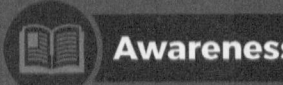 **Awareness**

- Awareness Videos
- Patient Education Videos
- Treatment / Procedure Videos
- FAQs

 International Patients

- Easy Call-to-Action
- Local Connect (if possible)
- Facility Tour
- FAQs
- Case Studies Specific to the Region
- Content in their Regional Language
- Testimonies Specific to the Region
- Complete Treatment Module Tour (Daywise Program)

 **Promotion**

- Camp Promo
- Treatment specific camp

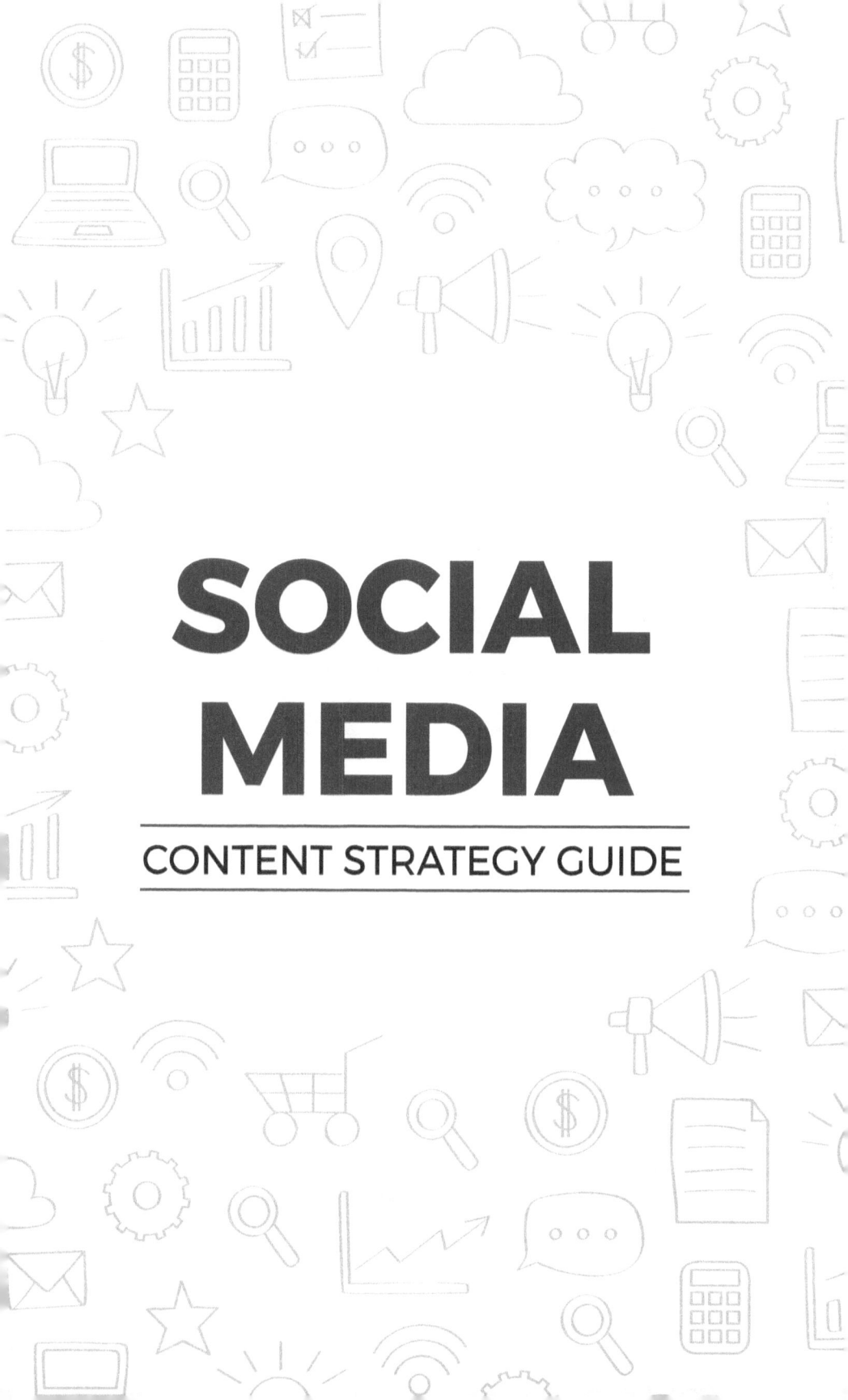

SOCIAL MEDIA
CONTENT STRATEGY GUIDE

Table of Contents

1. Establish Goals
2. Social Media Audit
3. Establish Your Target Audience
4. Competitive Analysis
5. Establish Brand Voice & Tone
6. Build Your Social Media Content Strategy
7. Social Media Marketing Measurement

Step 1:
Establish Goals

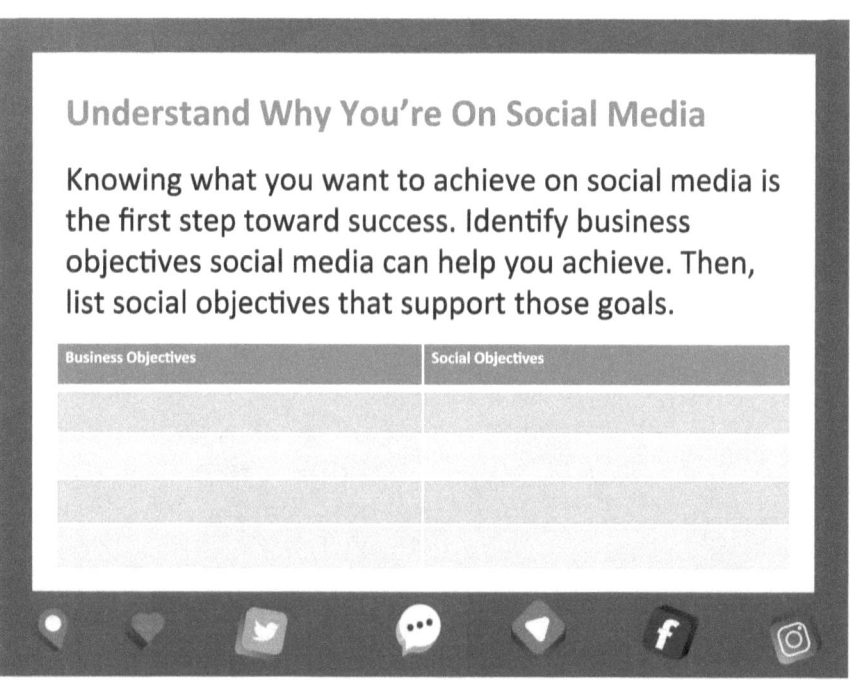

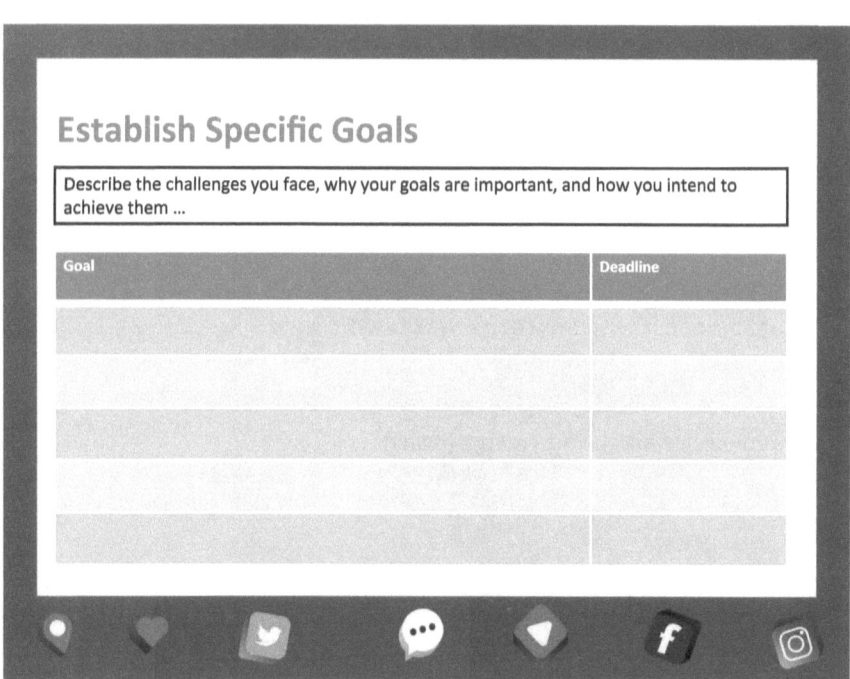

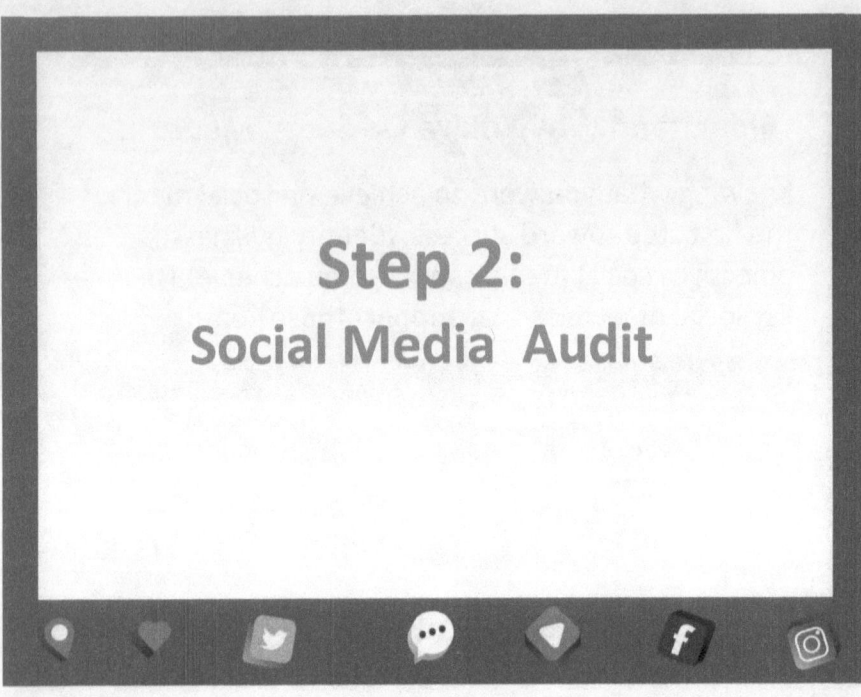

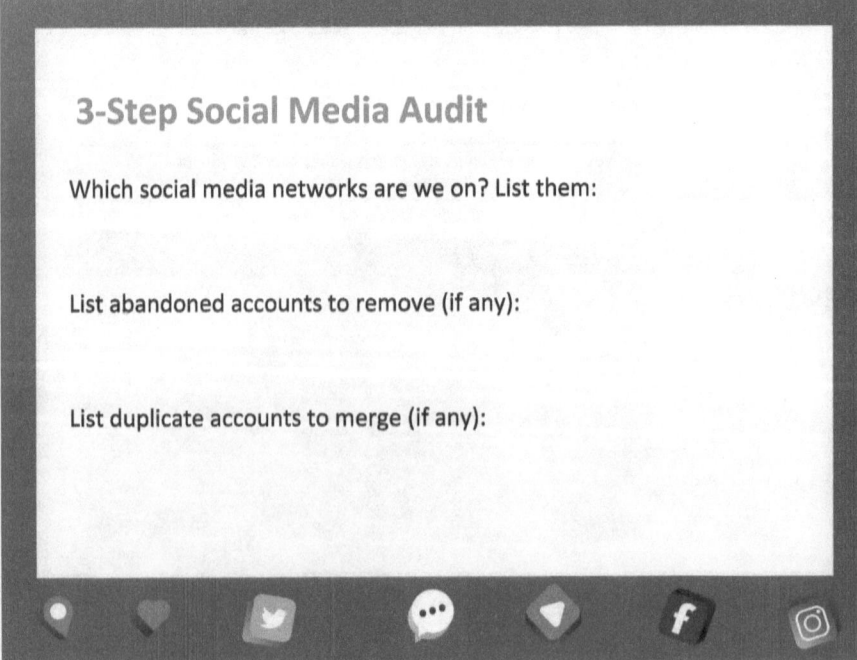

3-Step Social Media Audit

Which social media networks are we on? List them:

List abandoned accounts to remove (if any):

List duplicate accounts to merge (if any):

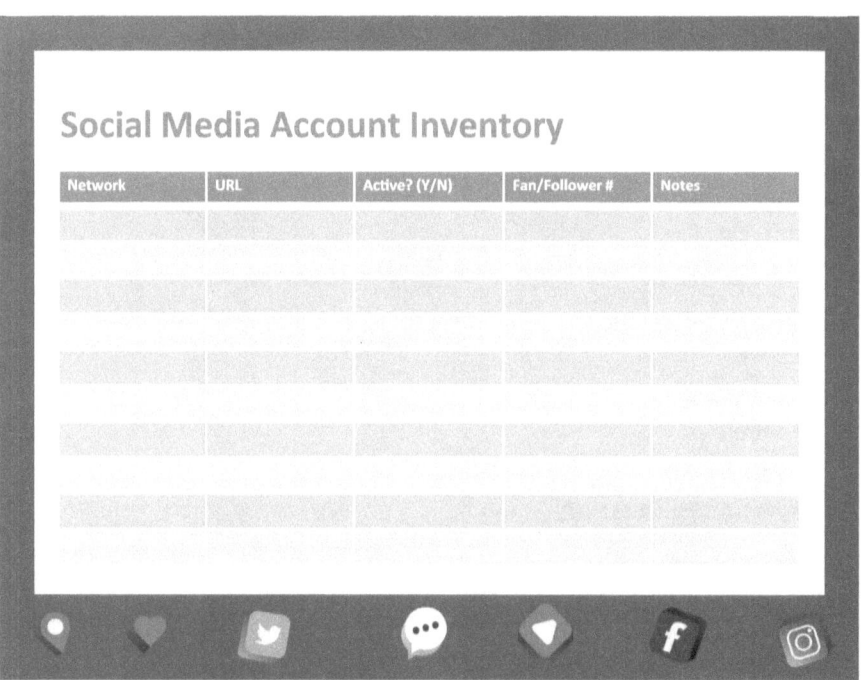

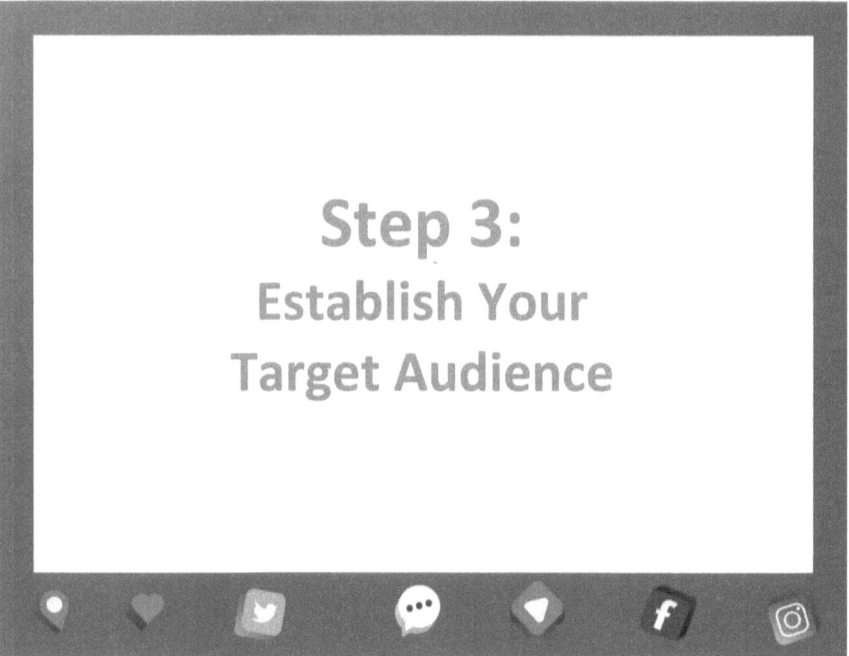

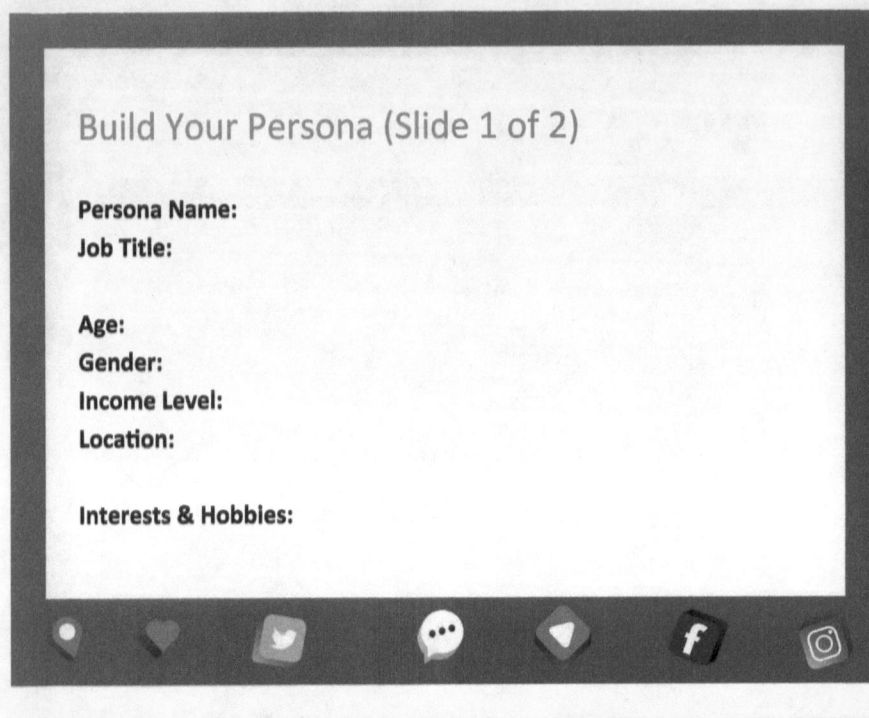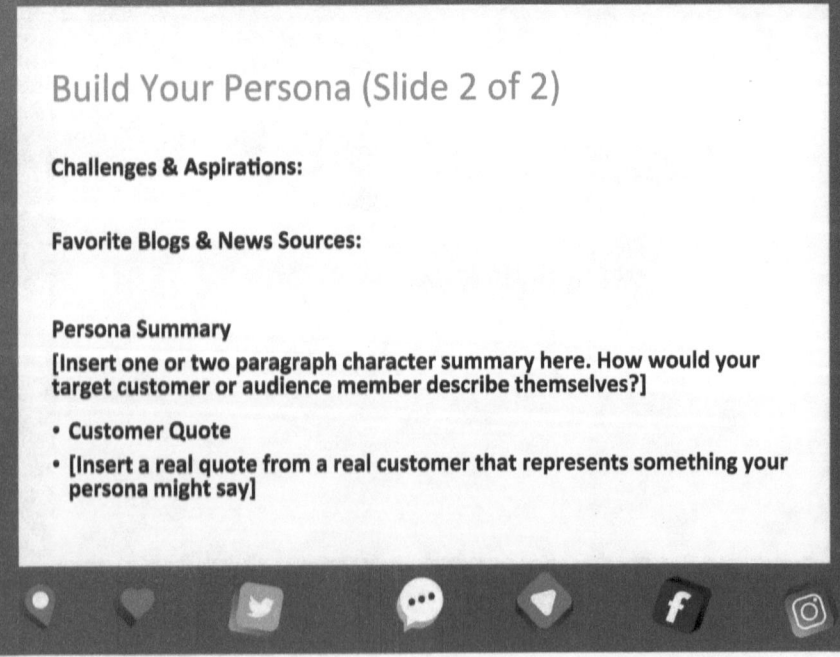

Step 4:
Competitive Analysis

Competitive Inventory

Competitor Name	URL	Notes

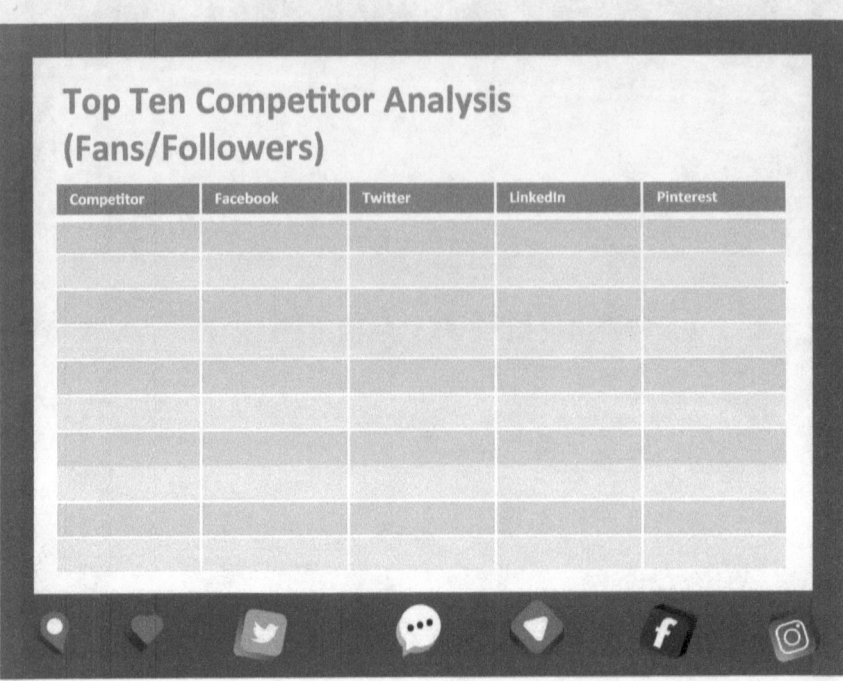

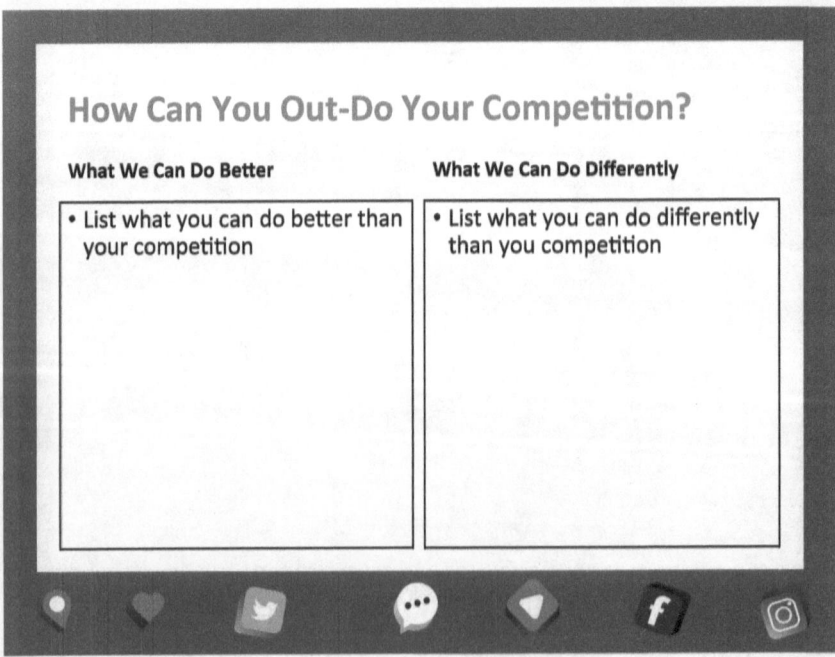

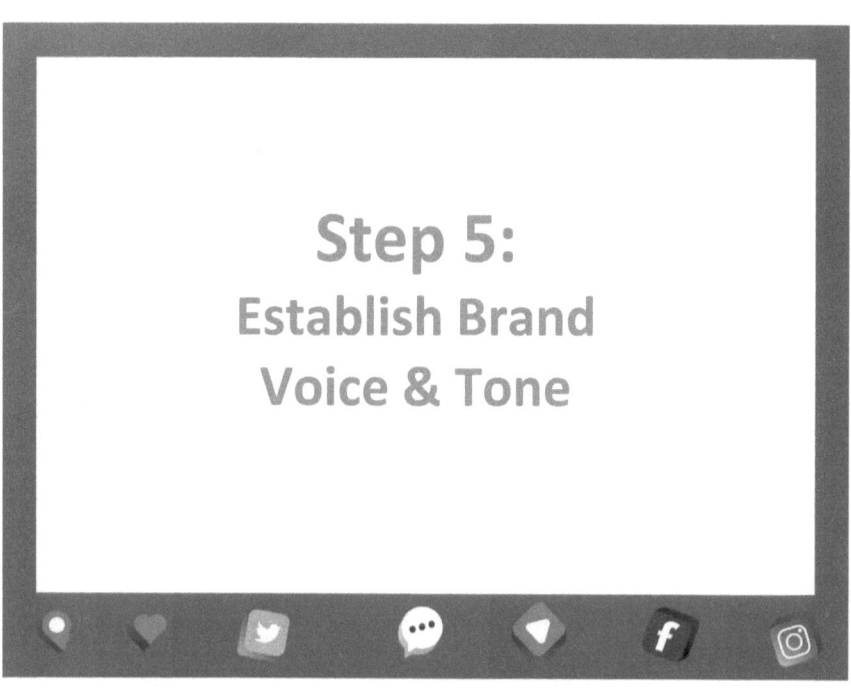

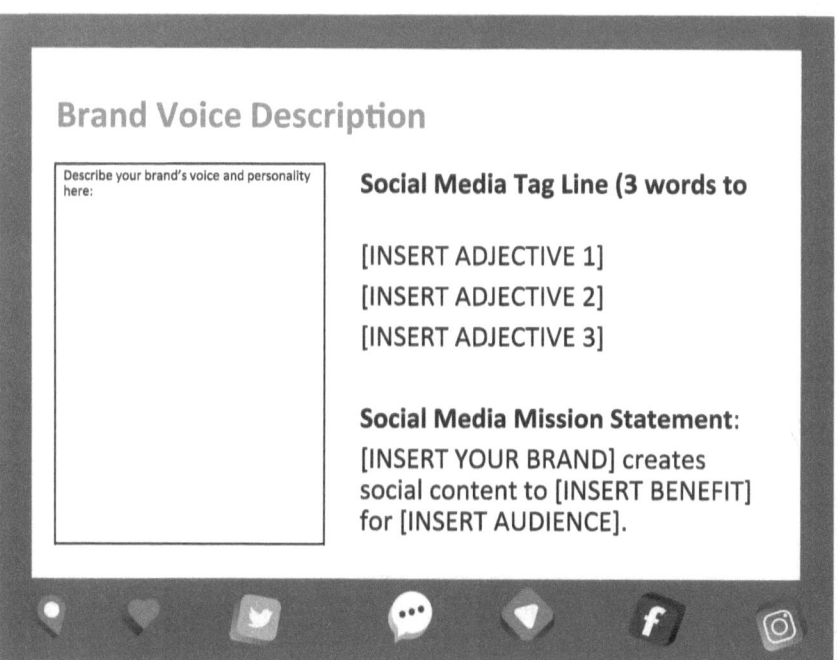

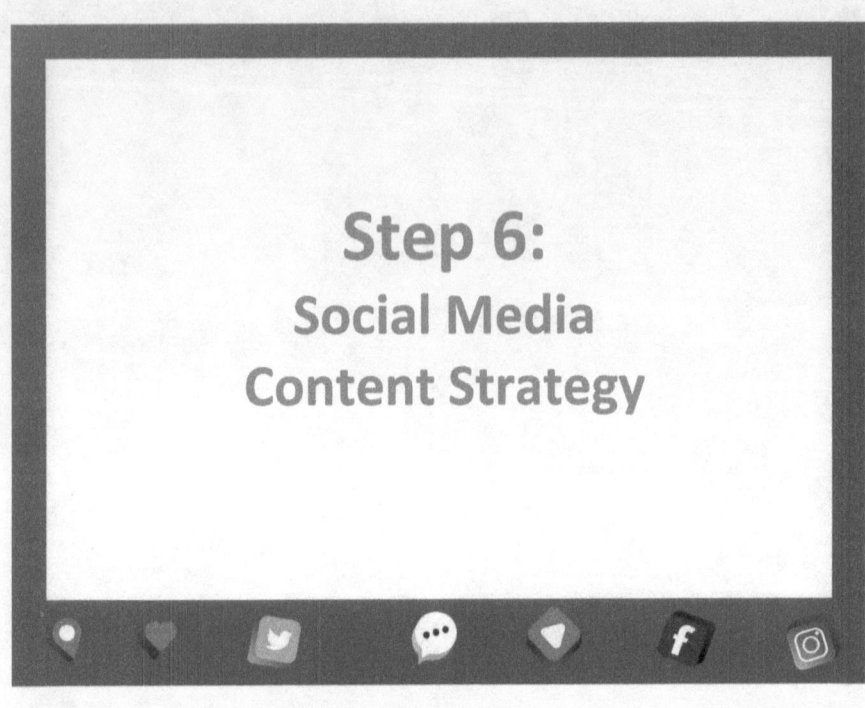

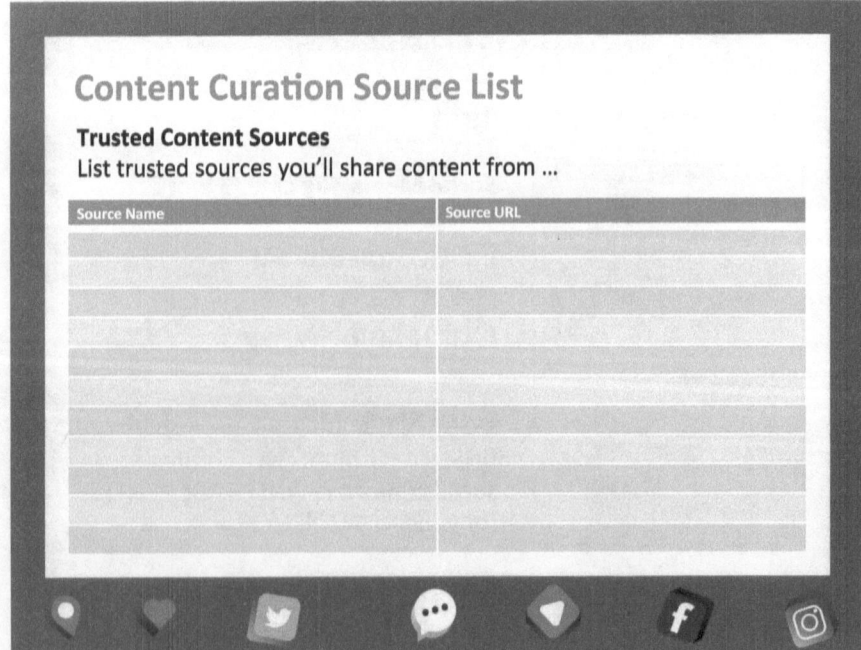

What Social Media Content Will We Create?

Content Types We Will Create:
List here ….

Content Types We Will Curate:
List here …

What Purpose Will Our Content Serve?

Original Content	Curated Content
[ ] Entertain	[ ] Entertain
[ ] Inform	[ ] Inform
[ ] Promote products/services	[ ] Promote products/services
[ ] Promote content (blog posts, ebooks, landing pages, etc).	[ ] Promote content (blog posts, ebooks, landing pages, etc).
[ ] Promote partners	[ ] Promote partners
[ ] Promote contests	[ ] Promote contests

Social Media Posting Frequency

Network	Posts Per Day	Posts Per Week
Facebook		
Twitter		
Pinterest		
LinkedIn		
Instagram		

Social Media Calendar Strategy

List upcoming events, product launches, and important dates to add to your content calendar:	Our content calendar will include:
[ ] [ ] [ ] [ ] [ ] [ ] [ ] [ ] [ ]	[Insert %] Original Content (Informative) [Insert %] Original Content (Promotional) [Insert %] Curated Content

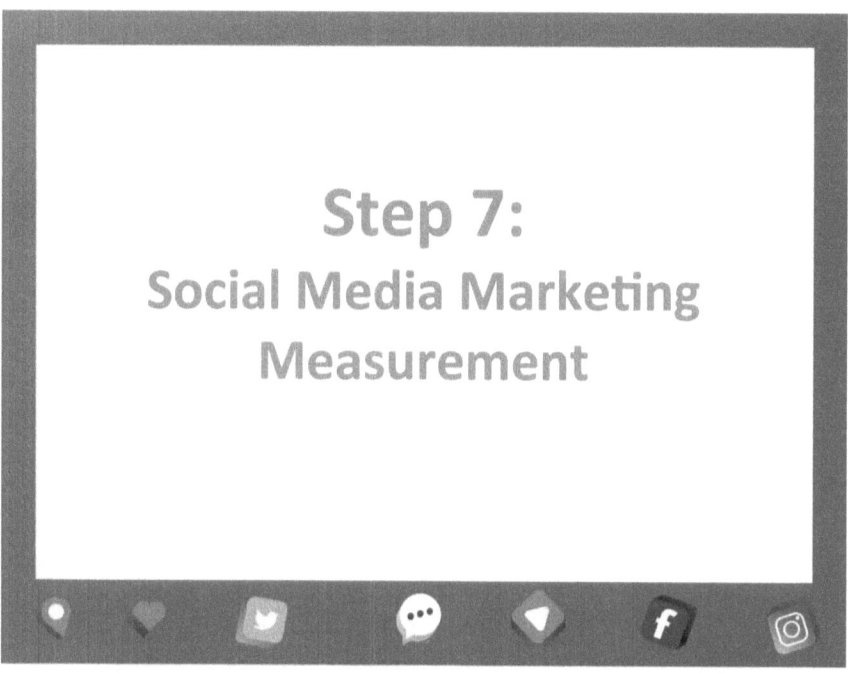

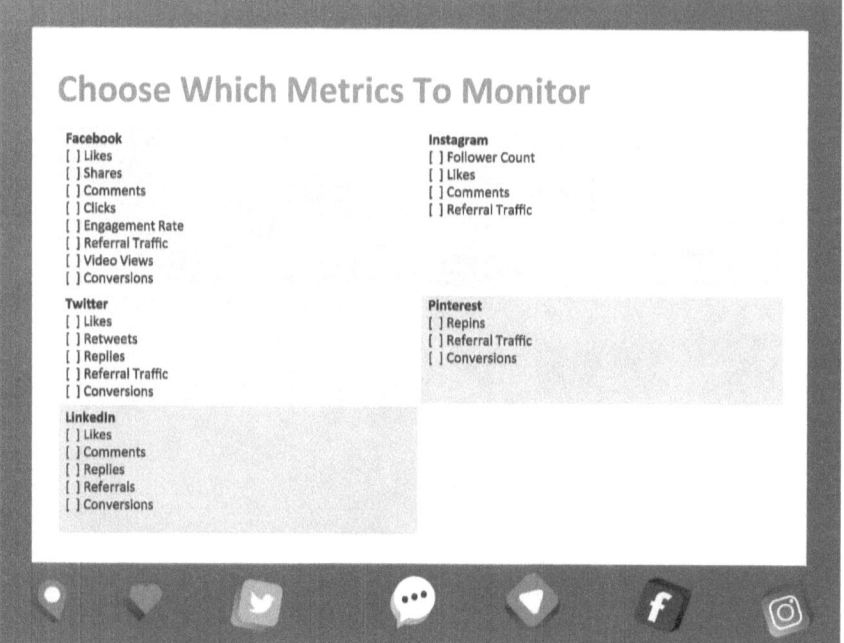

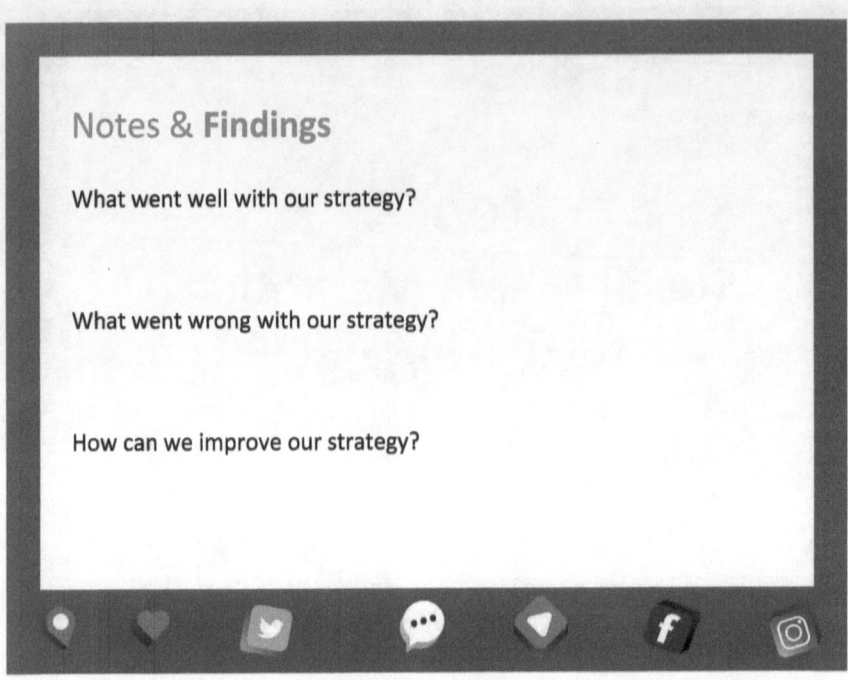

Notes & **Findings**

What went well with our strategy?

What went wrong with our strategy?

How can we improve our strategy?

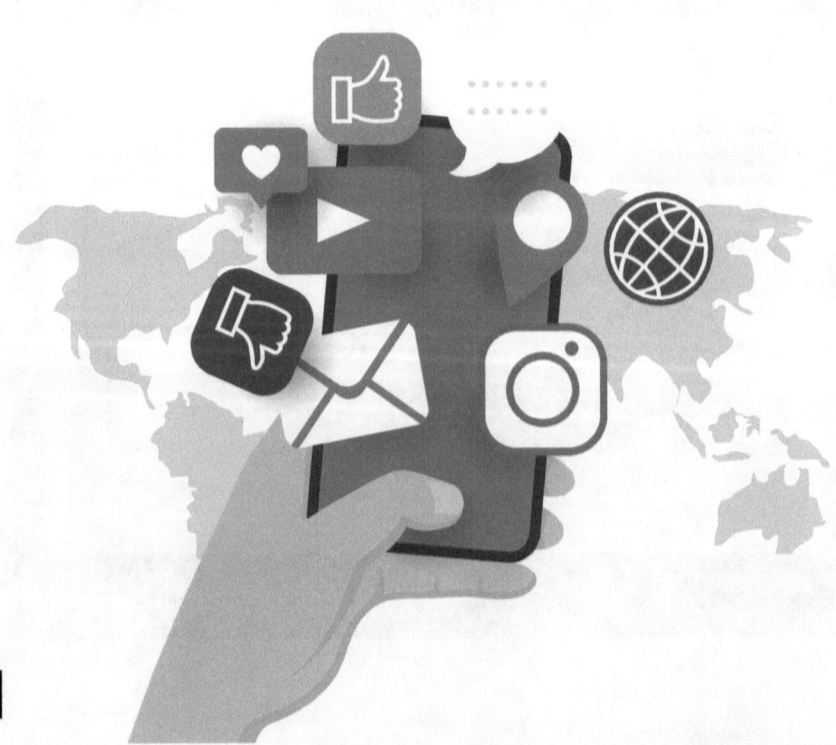

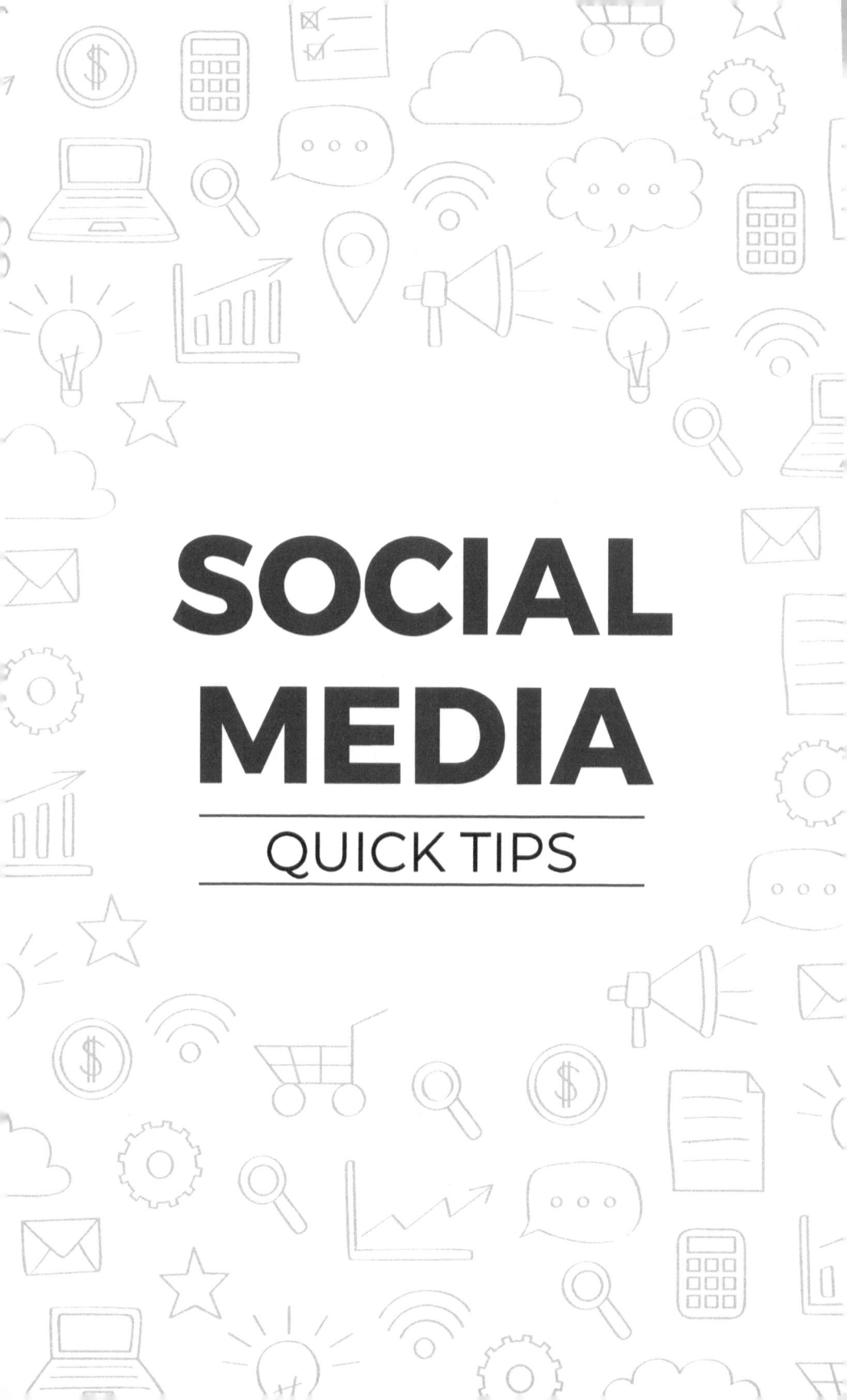

Types of content

Types of content to publish
Hospital Blog Posts
Posts Showcasing Your Hospital Culture
Industry News
Curated Content from other blogs
Question Posts
Awareness / Patient Education / Treatment Videos
Patient Testimonials (Text / Video)
Health Day Posts
Quick Tips And Advice
Memes or GIFs
Holiday Posts
Photos From Hospital Camps / Events
Post An Answer To A frequently asked question
Share Infographics (Mainly on Pinterest if you have audience there)
Start A Conversation With an influencer
Podcast Episodes
"On This Day In History" Posts
Hiring Announcements And New Team Members
Event / Camp promotion
Myth Busters - Q&A Live videos
Image Scrambles
Inspirational Quotes
Hospital Accomplishments / Milestones
Host A Twitter Chat
User-Generated Content
Share a Case Study On One of Your Customers
Share a Survey
Share a Fill-In-The-Blank Post
Reshare Your Top Performing Posts
Share Some Interesting Industry Research
Run a contest

Hot Tips

Make sure that your page name, cover pic and your profile pic should convey what your brand is about

Try 6 - 9 types of content and see what works

Instead of Posting 10 vague content just post 1 quality content

Pick social media channel wisely.

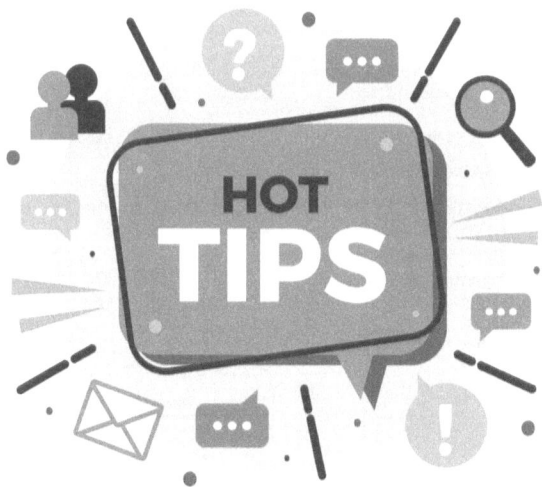

YouTube

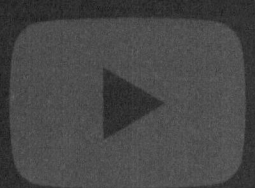

S No	Checklist
1	Conduct thorough keyword research and select the best keywords to target.
2	Optimise your YouTube profile, video titles, and video descriptions with relevant keywords.
3	Select video titles that describe the video and immediately grab attention.
4	Always add CTAs to your videos, descriptions, and in the "About" section of your YouTube channel.
5	Add website links in video descriptions and on your profile to direct traffic to your website.
6	Integrate with other social media platforms by using social media icons and links.
7	Leverage YouTube influencers to reach a much larger audience.
8	Cross-promote your YouTube videos on other platforms as well.
9	Optimise your videos, titles, and descriptions for mobile devices as well.

S No	Content that works
1	Any form of medium or long-form video content works on YouTube, as long as it is relevant to your audience and engaging.
2	Post Testimonial videos, Awareness videos, Steps involved in Treatment Videos, Short Motivational talk videos by doctors, Patient Education videos ..etc
3	YouTube is also a great platform to tell your brand story in the form of a video.

Instagram

S No	Instagram
1	Create and optimise your Instagram business account.
2	Use a profile picture that represents your brand, preferably your brand logo.
3	Use your bio to tell your brand story, describe what you do, provide contact details, and a website link.
4	Select a username that is recognisable and searchable.
5	Experiment with the different types of content like posts, stories, IGTV videos, and live videos.
6	Use popular industry hashtags in your captions to reach a broader audience.
7	Create your own brand or campaign hashtags to take your Instagram marketing campaigns to the next level.
8	Try influencer marketing and experiment with the different types of brand-influencer collaborations.
9	Leverage user-generated content from time to time and use tactics like featuring users in your feed to encourage them to create content for you.
10	Make use of Instagram's built-in analytics tool to understand what type of content works best for your audience.
11	Decide on a posting frequency and stick to your schedule.
12	Leverage Instagram Highlights to save important Stories and showcase them right at the top of your profile.

S No	Content that works
1	Instagram is a visual platform and therefore, high-quality, beautiful images are what will get you immediate attention.
2	IGTV and live videos can be used for hosting interviews and Q&A sessions.
3	Memes, GIFs, and other humorous posts also have a dedicated audience on Instagram. (This will work for any business)
4	Experiment with Instagram filters and the various video options like Boomerang videos, Superzoom, etc.

Facebook

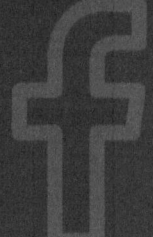

	Checklist
1	Create your Facebook business page and optimise it by selecting a good profile picture, name, and a compelling bio.
2	Ensure that you select the most relevant business category.
3	Create a custom URL that represents your brand and is memorable, instead of using the default URL.
4	Provide relevant business information on your business page, including your contact details and a website link.
5	Understand your audience by using Facebook Page Insights.
6	Use a chatbot to immediately greet and converse with any new page visitor.
7	Post regularly at the times when you're audience are online
8	Use Facebook advertising and create lookalike audiences to target specific sets of people.

S No	Content that works
1	Short video posts that are engaging and useful.
2	Posts with images work better than just text-based posts.
3	Use emojis to make your text-based posts stand out.
4	Experiment with live videos and stories as these are quite popular on Facebook.
5	Use Contests and use them in moderation
6	Bucket list posts — Fill-in-the-blanks
7	Funny memes
8	Share Content Created by Your Fans and Customers

Twitter

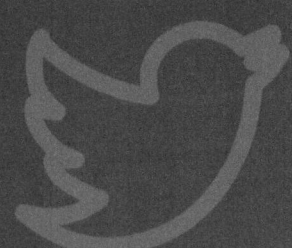

S No	Checklist
1	Though the platform has traditionally been a text-based, use images in your tweets to grab attention and make your tweets stand out.
2	Hashtags are your best friends when it comes to Twitter marketing. Find and use relevant hashtags to reach a much larger audience.
3	Optimise your Twitter profile by selecting appropriate profile and cover images and username.
4	Write an interesting bio describing your brand and what it stands for. Also, add your website link and links to other social media accounts.
5	Ask people to retweet, it doesn't hurt and might just get you more retweets.
6	Twitter is the best platform to engage in social media conversations on trending topics, so, comment, retweet, and share your opinions.
7	Mention relevant people or brands if you are sharing something related to them.

S No	Content that works
1	Short, frequent updates from an event or any latest happening with your brand.
2	Useful, informational tweets on trending industry topics.
3	Questions, quizzes, and polls.
4	Teasers or links to content on other platforms like your website.

LinkedIn

S No	Checklist
1	Create an impressive profile that helps you make a good first impression on your profile visitors.
2	Create a proper Hospital profile
3	Use keywords to get your profile to rank for relevant searches.
4	Leverage the power of LinkedIn groups and join relevant ones.

S No	Content that works
1	Informational articles on industry hot topics, case studies, etc.
2	Opinion pieces and thought-leadership content.
3	Reports, studies, long-form articles, etc.

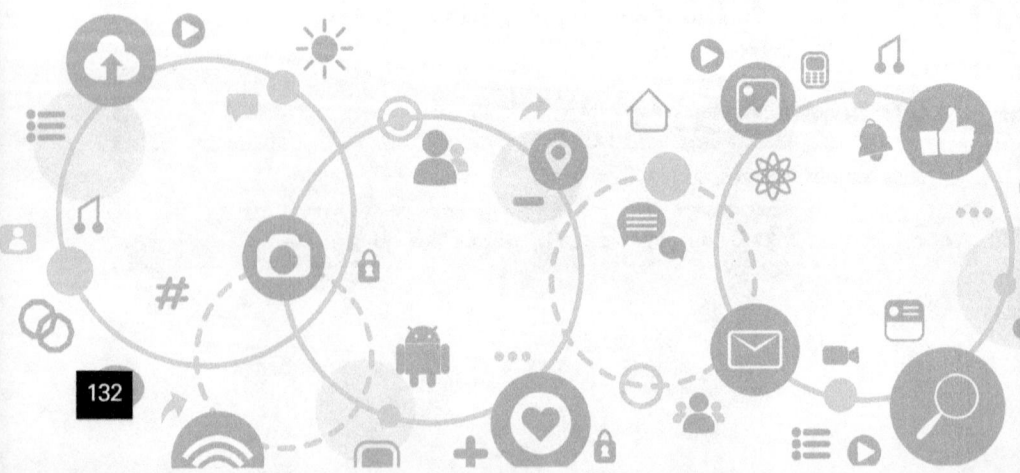

STRATEGY 7

"SUCCESS CREATES MORE SUCCESS, WHEN YOU MAKE SUCCESS REACH"

CASE STUDY MARKETING

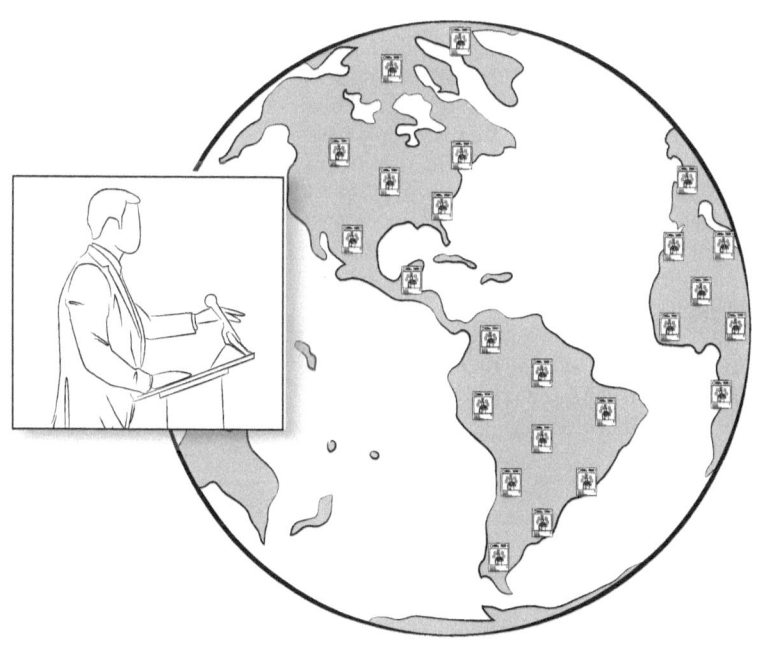

What is a Case Study?

A complicated case that is solved through the specialty-specific expertise of a specialist doctor is worthy to be called a case study. This can become a reference point for others to take inspiration from and act.

Why case studies deserve special treatment?

Case studies, when circulated, they give patients and doctors that unlimited confidence, as they are now aware of a way out of the same complication encountered before. A complicated case that made the patient see extremes in a night or two being solved smoothly by a doctor is a story that deserves the world's attention.

Effectively communicating your case study is important for you to not just talk about your expertise but the healthcare industry's capability as a whole. Whether it be a very rare unheard disorder, a geriatric patient delivering twins or a successful heart transplant in a just born and any other cases involving complications that deserves an ear from the world can give new hopes to people who are familiar with suffering.

Narrating such stories to the world has to be a task of pride as the end message can change each one's life in unique ways that you and I can list down. Yes, case studies are to establish one's expertise in solving that particular issue in that particular specialty. It's about the doctor and the healthcare brand who stood boldly behind the patient's life and took responsibility but it is also for those who have already given up and started counting their days. It is to push those who have left it to the almighty to try for one last time, and for all those doctors who constantly doubt their capabilities and limit their potential of touching lives and saving lives.

Extend the ray of hope through case studies; tell the world that there is not just light but a whole rainbow at the end of the tunnel.

7 Commandments of Case Study Marketing

1. They wouldn't know if you don't tell them

Case studies are treasures that talk for your experience and expertise, make sure you present them in the way people would want to. People want to know how big a difference you have created in somebody's life with your service. Also, a case study has so much new to introduce to this world. A case study caters more to compassion than anything else, it is to tell people that there is a solution to every problem no matter how big it is. It is to tell the world that an unheard complication can also be solved with hope and confidence as the primary instrument of cure.

2. Don't explain, narrate

The way your case studies reach is more important than how many reach them. Narrate the life-size difference you have made instead of saying merely before after stories. Include crucial changes the patient is enjoying after your service to make your case studies livelier.

Details don't matter if the stories don't reach. It is obvious that common people don't understand the crucial points and the nuances between life and death and everything in between that you handle on a day to day basis. Let these pain points in your profession be heard in a healthy way. Let your case studies express them.

Case studies have to be presented according to the end audience who is going to receive it, make sure the narrative is compulsive in expressing the soulful patient journey without many medical intricacies if it is going to be narrated to the mass. On the other hand, if it is going to be narrated to co-fraternity members make sure you have each medical detail & technical terminologies explained and enlisted along with the nuances of the patient journey.

3. Make each milestone count

The new height you have touched with your service matters big time. Each milestone in your career should contribute, especially to your profile's merit. Make them count by releasing a separate collection of your case studies. Such an initiative can make a difference in the amount of gravitas your healthcare brand has in the market.

Case studies should stand out from your other achievements as a medical professional. Make them that you narrate them with such gravitas and strength while preparing your profile.

4. Every complication deserves compliments when solved

A complication is one where many professionals have given up on the case, this really means a complication in the true sense. So, tell the world that you have taken a bold step and been at it successfully, without giving up, until the patient has fully recovered. The true purpose of taking that great step will be known only when the world applauds your infectious confidence in going that extra mile for your patient. There are days in your practice when you feel accomplished and you want to shout aloud from the rooftop channelize the momentary feeling and make it monumental by publishing a case study.

5. Be the inspiration and ray of hope

To bring out a case study means you have really done something that has made a difference to not just your practice and your patient's life, but has shown a new way forward to the whole world.

There are blooming practitioners who are looking out for that one boost of inspiration to hit them, serve the future generation with the right quality of inspiration to make the world a healthier place to live. Lead the way forward for other medical professionals to learn from you and create a legacy of their own. To create endless new beginnings for their patients who think they are nearing the end. Teach the world to value faith more than fate through your case studies.

6. Carry the beckon forward

Don't stop with just one. Having a case study out doesn't mean that that's the maximum you can get with impacting lives for the better. Teach the world with your case studies. Present them throughout in your CMEs and your other conferences that need people to narrate verifiable stories along with data and patient testimonial.

7. Grow from relatable to reliable

A healthcare professional need to be trusted to win new patients and the trust factor can be built only when people know how significant your service is. They wouldn't know if you keep them within your fraternity. Let your trust factor grow by itself.

The strength of your case study is directly proportional to the strength of your professional capabilities. Your case studies tell the world who you are and what you are actually capable of doing with all the right efforts.

The Case Studies that you collate must be documented properly so that they become etched in the books of your brand's legacy. They are a vital part of your career's milestone moments, Case Studies can become the defining moments of your healthcare brand as it is not just a solution, but a life-changing point for the patient and others to take great inspiration from them.

Pen down your case study today even if it takes time because it is worth it!

Note

7
CASE STUDY
ACTIVITY

How to compile a case study?

GATHER THE FOLLOWING INFORMATION

 Technical information: Facts and figures (with appropriate medical terms)

 Brief Patient History

 Patient testimonials (with consent)

 Derivatives from the case study

 Before - After photos

 Key moments that defined progress/ risk involved in the case

 References to any other similar complications ever come across in another case study

 Team involved in Patient Care

 Methods of practice you implemented

 Highlight the values of your organization that were reiterated

 Periodical meet-up with the patient to check on their status

 Patient with a motivational message to all others who lost hope

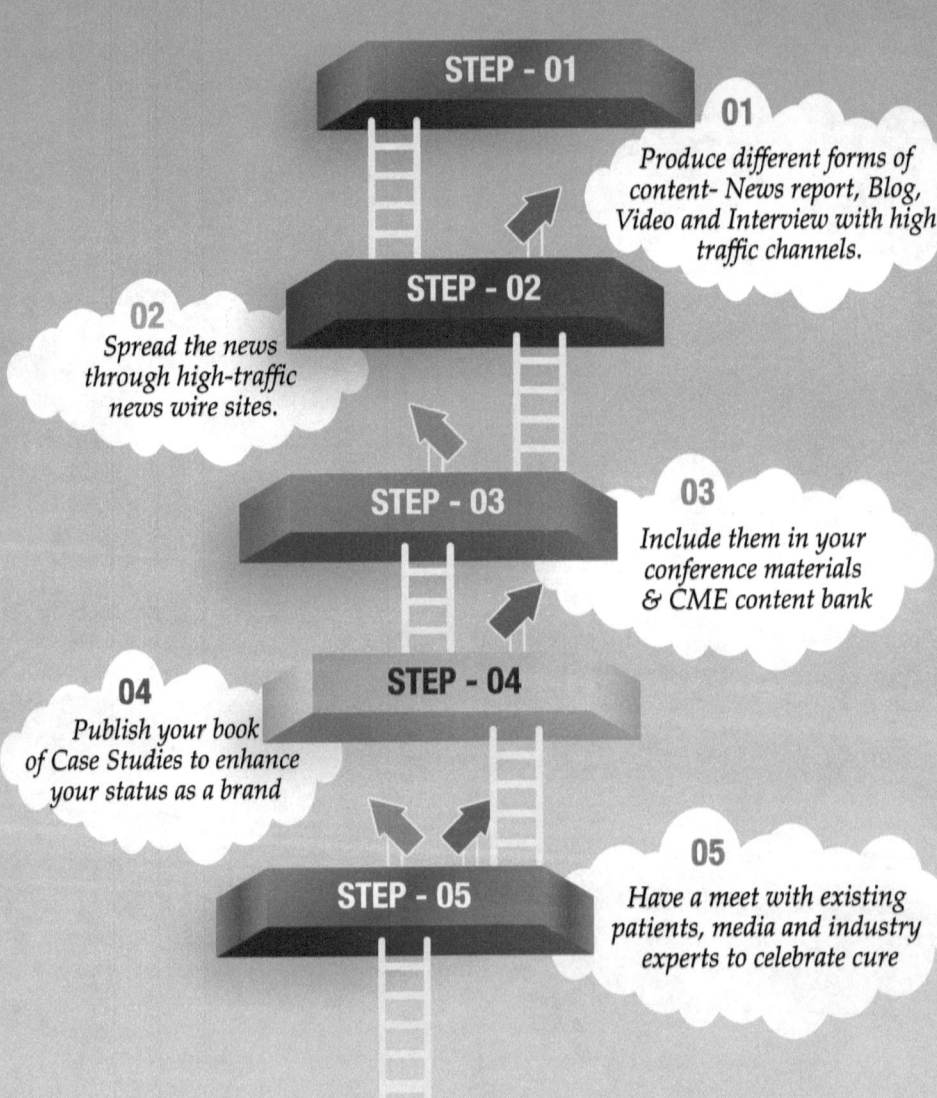

STRATEGY 8

"THEIR JOURNEY, DEFINES YOUR BRAND STORY"

PATIENT JOURNEY MAPPING

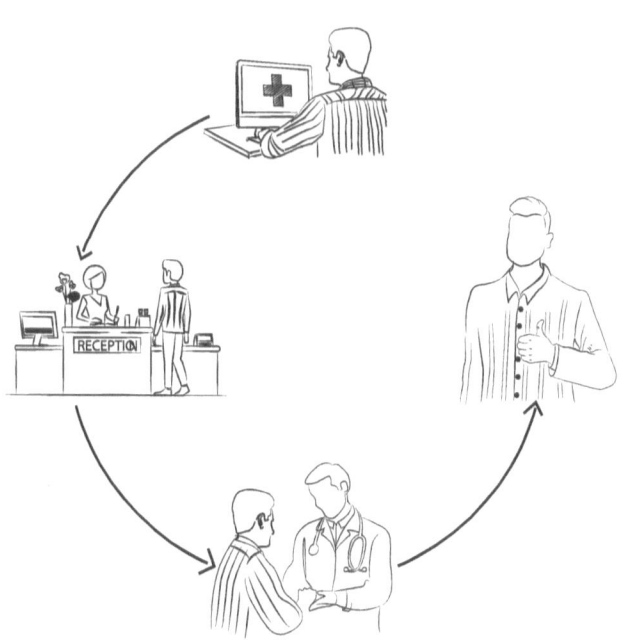

What is Patient Journey Mapping ?

Patient Journey Mapping is a major revealer of every hospital looking to cater to its own stream of patients. Tracking patient's journeys can be used to increase the ease of, and helping understand, what the personas can be. If you want to understand what kind of patients approach you for what and what is that one factor that is impacting your patient journey the most, then patient journey mapping will help you. Than being blindsided to what is flowing in and out of your hospital, take the full advantage of being able to measure and analyze. Thus, take informed decisions driven by data and pattern recognition of patient behaviors.

Patient journey mapping lets you understand what kind of people are approaching your healthcare brand, how they are being received by your healthcare brand and after reaching your hospital how they traverse through the whole journey. Patient journey mapping can tell you the effectiveness of your front office, waiting room patient touchpoints, non-medical staffs and all the other parameters that call for great importance in creating seamless patient journeys in your hospital.

Why Patient Journey Mapping ?

The more and more you analyze and study your patient journey, the more and more you will be able to touch on different types of patient personas. As deep as you know your personas, you will be able to logically classify them or profile them as per the in-flow trends, which indeed will help you crack the whole strategy to develop better methodologies to increase your quality of service. It will also help you to develop patient-centric new services, treatment packages and other seasonal healthcare brand updates as per the trends.

The entire process is the product!

Majority of the companies are becoming more conscious on delivering the product than creating the product itself, so the quality that your healthcare brand promises is not just about the treatment but about the whole process of providing that wholesome care from the moment a patient comes in contact with the healthcare brand until the moment patient is satisfied with the service. It's about the nuanced act of kindness as much as it is about the treatment or procedure. To patients little things matter and accurately mapping your patient journeys will tell you that little things are the deciding factors of a patient journey.

Now let me take you through the important aspects of patient journey mapping.

8 Important aspects in Patient Journey Mapping

1. Numbers never lie

Patient journey mapping reveals important data; it is the process that can fuel many other strategies that are deployed in favor of making your healthcare organization a strong one in terms of people management and retention.

2. Key to hassle-free patient experience

The more and more you understand your patient journeys the more accurate you'll get at designing them. The ultimate aim of patient journey mapping is to ensure that your patients and their guardians have hassle-free healthcare experience. It ensures that any patients' feedback or commendation, at every stage of their healthcare experience, is recorded and preserved for the welfare of the organization.

3. Use technology more efficiently

There are the latest software suites that are available that help you map your patient journey progressively. This, when used properly are the most efficient tools that can track patient journeys with zero manipulations and dysfunctions in data analytics. Gather appropriate information and data from these tools, which also helps in dashboarding for you to analyze them easily. Through this arrive at insights that may become epiphanies in making your healthcare brand deliver better care to your patients. Use analytic tools and charts based on the data collected to predict trends and mend the gap.

4. Best way to know and analyze your patient experience

When patient journey mapping is effectively implemented, you can infer something from every movement of the patient. Applying the inputs from journey mapping in your hospital increases the chances for a patient to form favorable opinion about your hospital and patient journey mapping lets you analyze the gap further . When you study your patient journey carefully you will get to know where you score high and where you score low this indeed will let you optimize operations inside your hospital and also upgrade it to patient's expectations.

5. Understand your patients more clearly

Patient journey mapping makes you look into your patient base more up, close and personal to find their needs more clearly and know their pain points more vividly. The patient's point of view in every step of the journey map will be visible with the trend that you observe. Their changing needs, behavior patterns, and other important traits help you better your operational quality.

Maybe your patients are looking for some very simple amenities that can be easily provided by your hospital but you are failing because you are overlooking them. Subtle things make a big difference to patients, even these can be studied through and rectified if you know your patient journey precisely.

6. Avoid patient leakage

When you cater to what your patient journey asks, you automatically upgrade your quality through which you will be in a position to deliver better care, ease out the patient's anxiety of going through the whole journey and also prove to be a perfectly hassle-free healthcare provider that you ought to be. Patient Journey Mapping spots all the gaps clearly through direct data points that your map reveals. Regularly updating patient touchpoints, scheduling follow-ups and rekindling the memory of their experience inside your hospital at appropriate periods may further prevent you from experiencing patient leakage.

Your patient journey map lets you analyze and tell your patients how better you can get with your promise and delivery. Through this, you eventually become that healthcare brand of aspirational quality. This lets your brand create more favorable patient journeys, in turn, creating favorable opinions. This is a sustainable strategy to reduce patient leakages.

7. Evidence-based way to cultivate a loyal patient base

Loyal prospects are a result of people, who are created through a meticulous process of regularly reminding people to keep a check on their health and living up to their expectations. It is one of the duties for your healthcare brand. Patient journey mapping tracks exactly this and helps in creating a database where you can follow up and convert them into your brand loyalists.

8. You v/s You: Learn, Unlearn and Relearn

Patient journey mapping lets you analyze the perks and pitfalls that your healthcare brand is enjoying among your target audience. Evaluate to increase the effectiveness of the process regularly. Every time you re-strategize the methodology of deriving insights from your patient journey map, you will get a new revelation, a new idea, a new problem to solve and a new reason to thank. So, use it to your advantage and compete with yourself, to better the quality of care you provide every day.

Now, is the right time, to start tracking your patient journeys if you aren't doing it yet. Track your patient journey map to become intelligent and responsive to the patient's timely needs. It is not you against your competitors, it is you against you. The treasure is not somewhere out there, it is very much within. If you understand your patient journey map well and make necessary amendments from time to time you'll carve a unique way towards your progress and prosperity.

Note

8

PATIENT JOURNEY MAPPING
ACTIVITY

IMPORTANT TOUCH-POINTS IN A PATIENT JOURNEY FOR EFFECTIVE BRAND IMAGE ACTIVATION

RECEPTION

The person at the reception is the first touch point and therefore sets the tone of the brand. Courteous / helpful / calm person wins the most

01

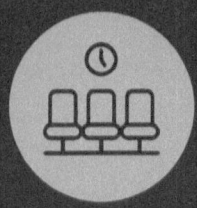

WAITING AREA

In every patient's journey the major part of it is spent waiting for their turn. So, the brand has to touch the patient's impression frame. So, internal branding and patient engagement through content is important.

02

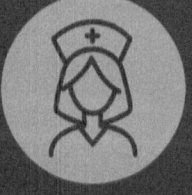

MEDICAL STAFF

In the journey they interact with the most crucial personality, the nursing staff. Qualities like resourcefulness, helpfulness, timeliness, and calmness are highly appreciated by patients.

03

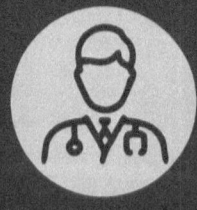

DOCTOR

The most important quality they expect from their doctor is that "they listen to my problems" and familiarity if they are existing patient. If the main hero sets the tone right then patient does not care about anything more.

04

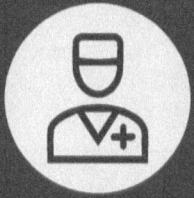

NON-MEDICAL STAFF

At times it may be required that the patients have to interact with non-medical staff for some support. Their discipline, helpfulness and resourcefulness is appreciated by patients.

05

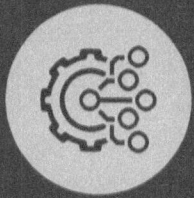

THE SYSTEM IN PLACE

How things get conducted inside an organization affects the positive mood of the patient about the brand. Hygiene, culture, technology in use everything matters.

06

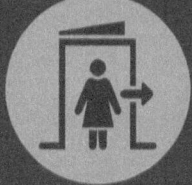

EASY & SMOOTH EXIT

At the time of discharge do patients get discharged smoothly without any difficulty. Does billing happen smoothly. How the send-off happens matters a lot in patient journey

07

POST PATIENT EXIT

In some cases the journey may continue even after they exit the premises if they would need periodic consultations or check ups. How the brand lives up to the expectation in each visit after that also counts.

08

The journey builds or breaks trust with the brand with every interaction at the touch point. Make sure every touchpoint builds trust with the brand much more deeply. A positively impacted patient who has had a smooth patient journey becomes your most effective WORD OF MOUTH agent who will refer to tonnes of patients to experience your brand forever.

Note

STRATEGY 9

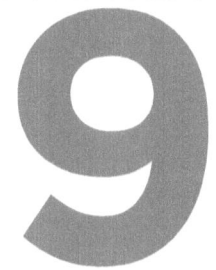

"LOOK BEYOND THE BORDERS, THE WORLD NEEDS YOU!"

INTERNATIONAL PATIENTS

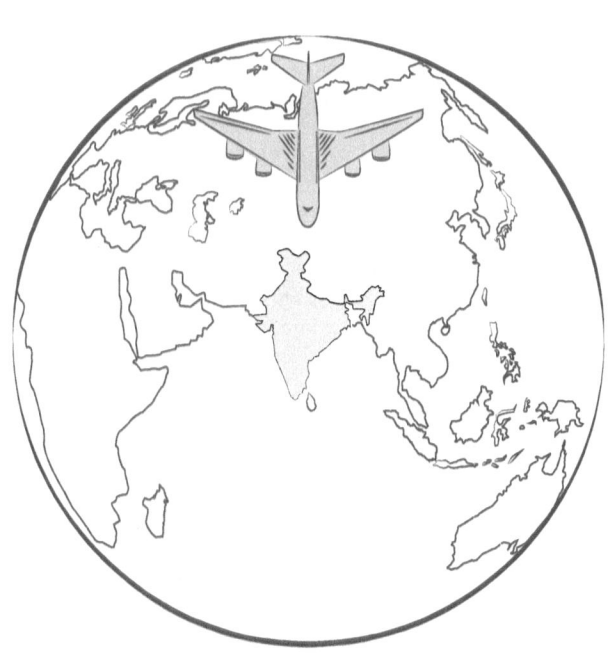

Serve International Patients

India exhibits a lot of impressive traits that make her a favorite healthcare destination and one of the most vital reasons for this is the quality and pricing of healthcare service.

Indian doctors, Indian Healthcare brands and Indian Medical Fraternity are growing stronger, day by day, to make India a sought after Healthcare Destination for international patients.

As a country, we are known for our hospitality and accommodative nature. The mere slogan "Athithi Devo Bhava" speaks for how well we want to treat our guests and tourists who come here. India, being an incredible destination for tourists from all over the world, has enough pull factors. Now the emerging boom of medical tourism proves that the healthcare industry has become one of the major pull factors, not just for tourism but also as a service exporter.

Hospitals are growing at a faster rate to accommodate and serve international patients, their infrastructural capabilities and their human resource capabilities. Any hospitals' idea of going global is friendly, for the industry' growth, and perhaps, the nations' growth. The number of patients traveling from other nations is increasing day by day. To take this culture forward, we need to nurture it through a structured process.

To direct international patient services in all the right directions and to reach the right doorstep of of those in need, at the right time, there needs to be a proper plan and a structured process of communicating with your international patients.

International Patient Marketing is a subject that the healthcare industry needs right now. With the boom of medical tourism, it is important that the healthcare industry thrives with the right kind of strategy that utilizes this opportunity and accelerates the scope of services to heal patients across nations.

11 Points to consider for Serving International Patients

1 Worldwide visibility makes anything a possibility

In this digital age, you can avail anything from anywhere, and so can your patients. Effective usage of the online medium can connect your healthcare brand to patients from any part of the

International Patients

world. In the touch of a button, you can connect to a patient from the farthest location you can imagine.

Having a great online presence for your brand is vital as people who need your service are worldwide; make sure your presence is strong. Now, it is easy for a patient from any location to find you and get treated.

With the advent of innovation in extensive telecommunication, going global for a healthcare brand is not difficult. If anything is stopping you from catering to medical tourism, then it is your own inhibition, inertia, and belittlement of capabilities of your healthcare brand.

2 Build a team with a shared vision

Build a team that is willing to go global. Ensure that your team does not deviate from the mission of taking care of international patients. A team that includes the right proportion of medical and non-medical staff is important if needed, hire staff who already have experience of dealing with international patients.

Make sure that every single hospital human resource that is interacting with the international patient directly, is trained enough on soft skills. More than plain language, orient them to their ethnic values and sensibilities to make them feel truly at home and reduce their stranger anxiety.

Make sure you have a group of patient coordinators who are multilingual and trained in handling patients from diverse geographies, understanding their inherent lack of clarity to the new journey they are on and comforting them into the hospital's atmosphere. To every international patient little things mean big. The nuances in ensuring their wellness are what will make their whole treatment journey a smooth one to be cherished with no fear.

3. Generate insights from trends in international patient journeys

Understand your international patient journey separately. Study their trends of a hospital visit, treatment journey continuation and other factors that could possibly affect the journey of an international patient. Strengthen the good ones and fix the hindrances.

Crack patterns in the kind of medical tourists that your healthcare brand is getting. Like every healthcare brand is unique, every medical tourist is also equally unique. They need to be given what they are individually expecting out of a hospital they are choosing. But, over a period of time, you would have gained the expertise to see a trend in your international patient in-flow.

See to improve your international patient operations by understanding such exclusive traits of patient journeys.

4. Patient coordinators are the result cultivators

Your coordinators are the key factors or touchpoints of your healthcare brand. They are the ones who travel with your international patients more than your medical staff. Patient coordination can boost patient satisfaction. The more clear and confident you keep your patient, the better it is.

It is not the communication skills or linguistic skills that matter in making perfect international patient journeys come true in your hospital. But the quality of your patient coordinators to listen to each international patient and give the kind of support they require.

Understand, that a team set to handle international patients is required to invest little extra efforts to empathize and understand the intricacies of their new environment anxiety and more, in order to comfort them properly.

5 Provide more than just the treatment

Patient packages just with details of treatment, procedure or prescribed diagnosis will go nowhere in satisfying your patient. Offer to tour your patient around your place that they can afford within the package, offer to provide their kind of food and other necessities.

India had been known for its rich heritage and tourist attraction spots much before medical tourism became a pull factor. So, more than the treatment, they need holistic solace for a wholesome recovery. Make sure you provide the same through your international patient service. Touring, getting some fresh air and getting to hear stories about the significance of our heritage sites are very helpful for a patient experiencing homesickness. All the more, they might recover very soon if they are given the best experience, both inside and outside the hospital.

6 Prevent yourself from restriction, kindle referral program beyond borders

Your practice should know no boundaries, practice beyond four walls. Believe, that the goodness your service creates should reach beyond what you see or think is your potential. Take the necessary steps to reach international patients who desperately need your service. Create a network through previous patients or trusted medical tourism networks or government bodies.

Make your referral program work from anywhere, anytime. Make your international patients your referral partners. Make your referral base strong, and not just in your own circle. A secondary referral network can be formed through your international patients and through the patient coordinators in that visibility radar.

7 Construct a chain to communicate the change

Construct your own channels to narrate the story in the best way possible. Bring the right set of people in the right way; make use of local and targeted channels to spread the significant case studies your service has created. Publish them in PR sites, social media platforms and other medical tourism sites targeting international patients to your advantage. Make sure you spread the goodness of giving the gift of cure to somebody who has crossed oceans for the same.

International patients need that "I am not new to this" feeling to go bold with their healthcare decisions and this can happen only when they hear several other success stories from their own country that matter. Break the boundaries and communicate the stories of touching lives and changing the lives of people beyond borders. People will know about your expertise and the strength that you have in your field only when you narrate your international patient case studies to the world.

8 Supportive Government Schemes & Airways

There are government schemes that reward you for serving people from other nationalities. Make sure you know and use these schemes to your healthcare brand's advantage. Get the nationwide recognition that your healthcare brand deserves. Get yourself registered with SEPC - Services Export Promotion Council, which will introduce you to new markets. Also, it will alert you on opportunities to expand your market throughout the world.

The Government body responsible for promoting the export of services from India is now taking so many special initiatives to cater to the medical tourism boom. SEPC is supportive of the growing healthcare industry, so they have special provisions that encourage each healthcare service brand to serve international patients under their radar.

Airways are expanding proportionally to the growth of medical tourism trends. With airports getting opened even in Tier 2 and Tier 3 locations, these locations will also enjoy the fruits of medical tourism. The expertise of healthcare brands from Tier 2 and Tier 3 doesn't reach international patients as much as metro cities because these healthcare brands do not reach them. So, unfamiliar destinations should be made online friendly to attract the attention of international patients who are searching for healthcare providers online. New airports are being planned in India and flight frequency is increasing for the nations from where patients are frequently traveling – all these are set to ease to-and-fro for international patients.

9. Narrate stories that matter

Narrate stories of agony to relief that you have created for your international patients. It is already an addition to your credibility that people fly across nations to access your service. Tell the world how significantly your service has changed somebody's life, of course, with their permission.

Narrate stories of how you cured that particular patient of that particular country and made a whole smooth patient journey come alive through your healthcare brand. Stories give people the courage, hope and confidence to not just choose your healthcare brand, but to choose to be a medical tourist without any inhibitions, hesitations or unwanted doubt.

10. Be transparent, accessible and available

Transparency in pricing is the first factor that gives your international patients the confidence that they are getting into safe hands. Let them satisfactorily enjoy the service by keeping them mentally prepared for the whole expenditure at each step. Keep them informed at each step. After the entire process is over, get their feedback and tell them you are available, even after they get back to their home, through telemedicine or online consultation follow-ups.

Give them the reason to choose you without leaving any gaps. Introduce them to the doctor who is going to treat them and also to the facilities that they will require during their stay at your hospital. The main factor that attracts and converts international patients to your healthcare brand is that how familiar and how reachable your healthcare brand is for those living miles away from you. Make avid use of technology to your advantage and go berserk at every international patient lead that you get.

11 Role of local facilitators

Appoint reliable local facilitators who will connect with your brand audience in those respective geographies. They will be able to clarify all their doubts in their language, about the travel and treatment. These facilitators will also accompany the patients when they are traveling to your hospital for treatment. The facilitators will coordinate on behalf of the patients with your in-house hospitality team for any needs and they will also make sure the patients understand without any doubt what the doctors say during the course of treatment, so that they can follow the instructions without any deviation during the recovery process. After the successful completion of the treatment, the facilitators travel back with the patients making them reach their home happy and healthy.

With a lot of infrastructural developments happening in India, it is the right time for your healthcare brand to venture into medical tourism. Use your service's potential to the fullest by serving patients across the globe with immense support from the government side.

Serving international patients is the best way to improve your brand awareness through case studies across markets. Also, taking a plunge into medical tourism by a healthcare brand is not a very big step to think and take. If you are confident about the quality of service you provide and the kind of infrastructure you are offering your patients, then you are all set to invite international patients.

Take one step at a time. start by having one international patient through a reliable channel and serve them big on every aspect they want to be served, to see the real effect of your service helping somebody completely stranger to you. Don't restrict the scope of your service, remember the whole world needs you.

9
INTERNATION PATIENTS
ACTIVITY

International Patients are looking for specific communication in your website and those are the below

1. Easy Call-to-Action
Whatsapp / Phone Number / Email / Chatbot

2. Local Connect
If you have a local facilitator for follow up it helps. Share the local connect on your website

3. Content in their Regional Language
Make them feel you are already close to them.

4. Build Specific Pages for each geography
You can add relevant content in their regional language

5. Testimonies Specific to the Region
Pick & Highlight testimonies from the same region. So that they can verify & build trust faster.

6. Case Studies Specific to the Region
This is another important ingredient to help them know complex cases you have already handled

7. Facility Tour
Give them a Virtual Tour of your facility. Patients are very particular about your infra capabilities and wont come to you if you have a poor setup

8. Complete Treatment Module Tour
Give them a plan of what will happen from the day one of their travel till their safe return to their homeland.

9. FAQs
Have a dedicated FAQ section that helps them get answers to all their queries.

4 WAYS TO ACQUIRE INTERNATIONAL PATIENTS

Online Marketing
You can market through Google adwords and Facebook, targeting those respective geographies

International Medical Fair
Participate in International Medical Tourism Fair
You can interact with patients directly in some fairs and also recruit local facilitators

Invite Facilitators to Your Hospital
You can also sponsor the trip of facilitators who have promised to send business or shown interest

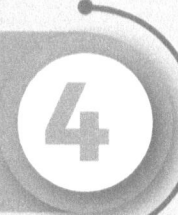

Tie-up with Govt /International Hospitals
You can tie-up with other government health offices / hospitals / doctors who refer patients to get treated abroad

Note

STRATEGY 10

"REDEFINE YOUR TARGETS, REDEFINE YOUR MARKETS"

REBRANDING

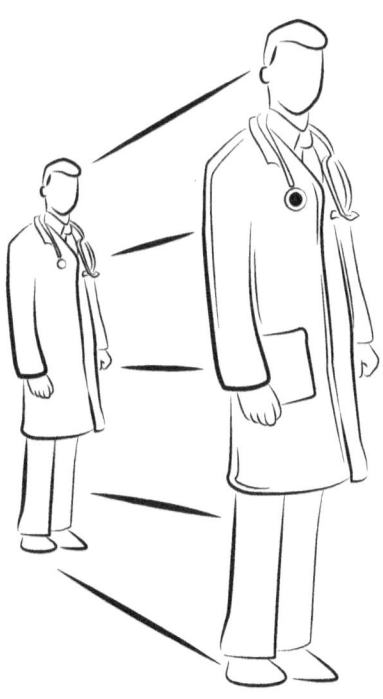

Rediscovering who you are on a time to time basis is vital for staying relevant and in demand. Every healthcare brand stays in relevance with its patients through by regularly redefining their approach in getting nearer to their potential patients. The near future of your healthcare brand will take a redefined new flow to resonate more with your potential patients.

Rebranding is the process of communicating your exact brand message and promise that persists today through channelized efforts and well-thought strategies. There is an unintentional impression that every brand leaves behind through the word-of-mouth that it generates through people near and dear to the brand. This may work in favor or against to the brand, but well-arrived rebranding efforts for a brand can make the biggest of difference to it positioning.

Over time, there is a need, that the brand communicates accurately and openly, to form a desirable image for itself that maximizes the brand's potential in reaching out to people and becoming a healthcare brand close to their heart. This does not imply that rebranding is purely about communication, it is also a process where a brand has to undergo a change from within.

Changing the healthcare brand's DNA from within with respect to what it may call for .

11 commandments of Rebranding

1. Stay in line, Stay in focus, Stay in demand

Rebranding helps you to catch your potential patient's pulse and stay tuned with it, to reach them without a communication gap. People today want to stay updated and upgraded and they prefer their healthcare brand also do so. Being updated as someone who decides on the brand is as important as keeping the brand itself updated. Applying rebranding techniques to your brand can be very prospective if they coincide with the tastes of today. Revisit brands that are known to be iconic in nature, you'll also notice that they have reinvented certain elements of the brand over time.

2. The approach should change as the needs change

Brands, to stay forever concurrent, need to commit to a very challenging exchange between themselves and the marketing environment. It is the need to give up on the stubborn, unproductive traits of a brand and adapt to the need of the hour. It does not mean that all brands may have to succumb to fads that the target group put forth, but they have to stay relevant.

3. Make yourself matter, every day

Every day there are enough opportunities for every brand to craft their image carefully in the mind of the patient. Make yourself matter on a day to day basis by taking your brand engagement on a level higher than it is. Use different channels, different mediums and targeted tonality of communication, as the day demands.

4. Talk to them in today's terms

Talk to them in the updated lingo, catch climates of opinions like prevailing patient fears and expectations of a healthcare provider and then deliver accordingly. Treat your patients to the standards that the globalized world has set.

If a patient expects a particular brand to address or come forward with their take on a globally trending topic, let your brand do it. This a major way that every classic brand stays youthful.

5. Your brand should mature, not age

A brand, budding or established, needs to set right the way in which it would like to evolve. Great healthcare brands gracefully pass through years of achieving high-level patient satisfaction by reinventing their style and standards according to the need.

6. Rediscover; yourself, reinvent your success formula

Even a century-old brand needs a breath of fresh air. It is important that you should also see that you analyze the market trends and gaps and re-tweak what your brand strategy is, to see unshakable success. If a very popular brand has been known for its maternity care, now, its target audience would want to avail fertility services too. So, reworking your service and offering along with the soft traits of your brand is important.

7. Be deep-rooted by values

While you are deep-rooted to the base of strategic values your brand was built on, you should also take ardent care that you don't become stagnant on one section of your target patient base. Make yourself available and appealing to your patients across generations. When it comes to healthcare brands, there is a traditional pattern i.e. when people invest their trust in a healthcare brand, they aggressively recommend it to the generations to come too. Ironically, the desired customers of some brands change, but the brand does not. Here is where brands that are not properly rebranded seem to lose out. Being relevant has to be a part of your values.

8. Do not be afraid to reinvent yourself

It is obvious that your present status reached some far and carries its own value, but how far can they sustain and sound relevant, irrespective of ongoing trends? This is the question that you need to answer to take unbridled steps to reinvent yourself. Reinventing a brands most crucial parts can put you through self doubt, but that will eventually wither away. All that will remain is a reinvented brand that everybody will look forward to.

9. Reflect the change within

Make sure that your urge to rebrand is not out of an impulse or the pressure to match up to your competitors. It should be a result of intra-organizational development and organic evolution of your brand. Understand, that with time, all brands change and this can be leveraged to advantage. When this natural process occurs as your brand ages, notice how your USPs change and capitalize on them.

10. Re-craft a stronger identity to re-instill your legacy

The maturity of your identity and the strength of its representation changes according to time and age, or by the markets normalized standards set by your competitors. Reassure your patient base that you are in it to win it. Win more patient loyalty and patient trust by rebranding. The act of rebranding is comparatively easier to adapt to, than making that reinvented brand stay strong with your target audience.

11. Your rebranded self has to be communicated

Appoint reliable local facilitators who will connect with your target audience. Brands evolve over time and that evolution grows with its target audience. But when the brand consciously undergoes a phase of renaissance, then it calls for a new communication targeted towards its brand loyalists. Be it a small change or a huge makeover of brand image, both have to get to the audiences' ear promptly. Any brand updates have to be informed properly to its people.

Rebranding is a conscious process of transformation that every brand has to go through at some point in time. All brands should periodically audit and renew their presence amongst the target audience. When there is a mismatch, deficit or, if anything can better then, rebranding can be the right solution to restart.

Note

10
REBRANDING
ACTION PLAN

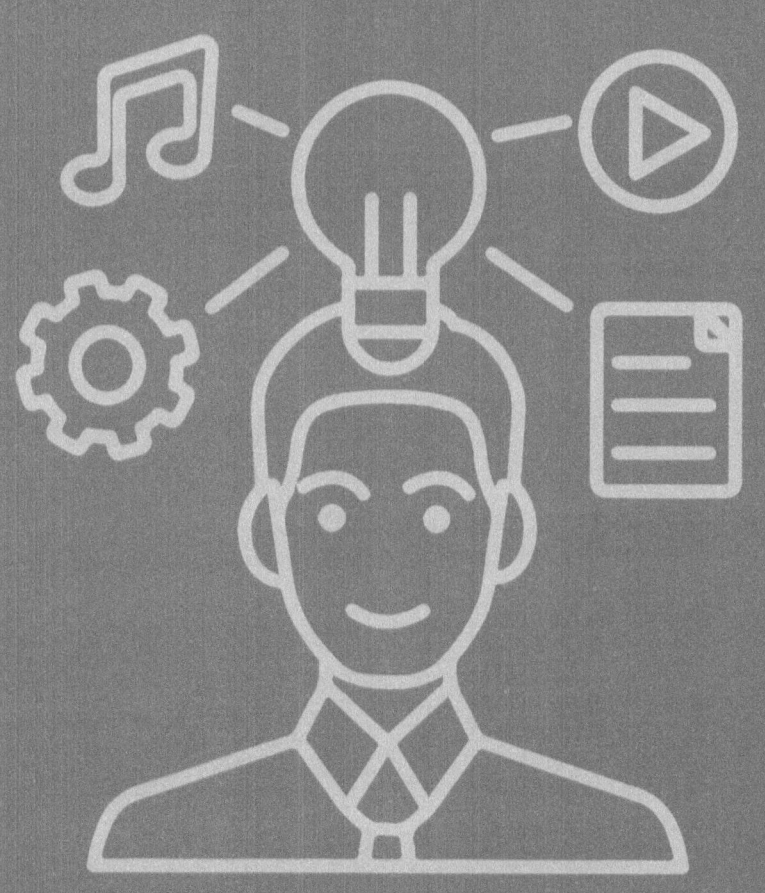

ANSWERS THESE QUESTIONS ON REBRANDING

Q. Over the past years, what is the most evolved characteristic of your healthcare brand that has to be communicated today?

A.

Q. What is that one sole purpose behind your rebranding move? Is it just to say you still exist or have you reinvented your purpose?

A.

Q. If there is one thing that makes your present brand outdated, what is it? HOW would you like to change it?

A.

Q. Who are your new set of target groups and what you found new in your existing audience?

A.

Q. What are the elements you would like to retain and what are those that you want to eliminate?

A.

ANSWERS THESE QUESTIONS ON REBRANDING

Q. When is the last time you felt that your brand and the present market climate has a gap to be bridged? Why?

A.

Q. Has anything typecasted your brand? Do you think your brand is much more than that one trait?

A.

Q. What would you like for todays' patients to think about your brand?

A.

Q. What kind of a campaign do you think can evoke a new image in your target patient's mind?

A.

Q. What are your goals after the process of rebranding?

A.

STEP BY STEP PROCESS FOR REBRANDING

UNDERSTAND YOUR POWERS & WEAKNESS
Understand the inherent brand powers and the weakness. Understand how you can amplify your powers and curb on your weakness.
01

DEFINE YOUR REBRANDING MANTRA
Understand by rebranding what is the change you are going to bring inside and outside to your brand. Arrive at the rebranding module that should encapsulate these changes.
02

ARRIVE AT REBRANDING COMMUNICATION
Now arrive at a perfect communication that talks about your rebranding - with new focus and old values.
03

COMMUNICATION AT WORK
The rebranding communication should make employees more proud about working for the brand & build loyalty. Existing / lost customers should get new lease of hope, new prospects should relate to the positioning well and stakeholders should find confidence.
04

TEST IT
As rebranding is like giving life to the slowly dying, any mistake could be highly disastrous. So, test the communication with a closed group of audience- see if they are able to relate to the message and then explode it
05

SPREAD THE MESSAGE
Spread the message through the online and offline mediums also, make sure your brand marketing collateral and every bit of your brand that carries your brand logo carries this. Give due importance to internal and external hospital branding in communicating this change.
06

LIVE THE PROMISE
When people want to experience the brand, they will want to check if you are true to your promise. So always make sure that you create systems in place that deliver well on customer satisfaction. Every satisfied customer is just not one, but has a power to influence a million.
07

STRATEGY 11

"BY MAKING OTHERS WIN, YOU WIN BIG"

COLLABORATION

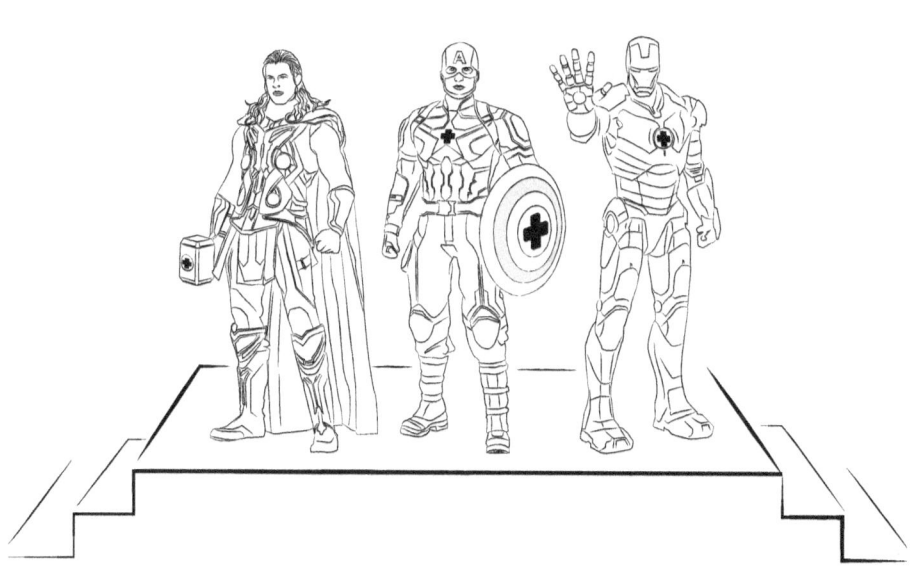

Collaboration - The Need of the hour

Collaboration guarantees additional strengths, added and advantages coupled with collective growth and success. In the healthcare industry, multiple factors decide a hospitals well being and human resource is one such crucial factor that decides how much strength you can collectively gather to thrive in the ever-increasing patient & market demands. No organisation can say that they have enough right resource, always there is a demand for the right resources and all these expert resources who are instrumental for success and growth can be hired or partnered when your plan for the mutual growth is clear.

Collaborate, but do not compete with specialisations and super specialisations in a given specialty. it only makes sense that you collaborate with a specialist within your fraternity to pursue and keep yourself engaged in those micro specialisations, and collaboration can do that for you.

Also, interesting collaborations are fostered through Continuous Medical Education. There are a lots of specialists today who are increasingly getting into hands-on training, which, in a way increases the skillfulness of fellow practitioners on one hand and the other they get engaged in handling all the complex cases, which are referred by their students. They create a teaching and learning community that constantly gets into skill up-gradation, research and and inspiring others to pursue a super specialisation. An environment filled with teaching, learning, research and continuous skill up-gradation is an excellent implementation of collaboration as a core principle, where there is no imaginary fear of competition. There is only mutual respect, recognition and overall development, which is in favour of the organization, fraternity, and patients.

Key aspects of Collaboration

1. Put your patients first; partner with the caregiver they need

Collaboration has become the key to satisfy patients of all kinds. Realize that the main aim of your hospital is to put patients and their needs first, so satisfy them by bringing resources from any fringe. So, always have a list of partner caregivers who can support your patients at the time of need and be available to help you.

2. Don't struggle for talent, strive for a treasure of partners

If you are looking to hire an experienced specialist for each department, then maybe it is not going to be as easy as you want the process to be. In some cases, hiring would be very expensive and may not be right; in such cases partnering would be the right method of collaboration. You can provide the infra and the expertise can come from the specialist for which there can be mutual agreement on revenue sharing.

3. Share your strengths to see comprehensive results

In a hospital, it is always a team that solves issues for the patient, more than an individual. Strength, as a team of practitioners and non-medical staff is unmatchable. Use the competencies of different professionals at right times to see results that satisfy a lot more parameters. If infra is your strength, share that strength with a specialist who may not have the right infra to support their patients, but may have the expertise. By making your infra open, you can make optimum utilization of capacity which is very much needed for the smooth running of your hospital. Collaborations like these are also very much welcome.

4. Expand your market share

Unleash the fullest potential of your market share by collaborating, so you will enjoy the greater part of the pie by serving more in need. Growth becomes faster when people with expertise find reliable brands with great infra support come together. Through this collaboration a lot many patients can find a ray of hope. The collaboration should aim at helping people through the right diagnosis and transparent care in numbers, which can significantly reduce the cost for both the collaborators and patients. The end result should be enjoyed by the patient who has to pay less by enjoying quality care.

5. People prefer a one-stop solution, do you have it all?

People, once they like to associate with a healthcare brand and start trusting, don't want to take chance with another. They will want to learn that what are the other services that provided which they may need. People want all their healthcare needs to be solved in one reliable place, if that can be possible. It is only natural that one healthcare provider cannot have it all, so, collaboration is important not only for growth, but also to compensate inefficiencies of each other which cannot be solved without effective partnership. The patient journey becomes much smoother when a patient can find the required service in the place they trust.

6. Hire specialized experts for allied healthcare operations

There is a lot that a hospital requires more than the hospital itself, like hospital management software, ethical marketing strategy, hospitality partner and others. So, invite healthy collaborators to partner with you to run your organization seamlessly. These partners will help you in bringing operational efficiency within the organization and will also help in effective outreach communication about your care stories which people want to know more about.

The evolving world needs evolved organizations that are smart enough to collaborate and use resources efficiently. It does not make sense to invest heavily in infra for everyone, it will ultimately lead to unethical practices just to recover the investment cost. Instead, growth and success can be achieved by doing smart investments in places where it is required and other essentials can be used through collaboration. There can be a common infra investment done by people in a particular geographical region and it can be used by all others on the use & pay model which can itself become revenue stream for investors and can bring costs down effectively to patients, this is another beneficial collaboration model. You can evolve your own collaboration model of your choice as long as the basics are followed which is providing seamless affordable patient care.

11
COLLABORATION
ACTION PLAN

COLLABORATION
STEP BY STEP PROCESS

STEP-1: UNDERSTAND WHERE TO COLLABORATE
Understand in which area collaboration really necessary, by collaborating what is expected to happen.

STEP-2: UNDERSTAND WITH WHOM TO COLLABORATE
Short-list the candidates or brands that would be appropriate fit for your brand for collaboration and evaluate on paper the impact of each collaboration before telling them.

STEP-3: UNDERSTAND ON WHAT TERMS TO COLLABORATE
You can have standard terms for collaboration but in most of the cases wherein your collaborating partner brings in enormous value then you may have to settle on mutually beneficial terms. Have a written agreement with exit policy clearly defined.

STEP-4: UNDERSTAND WITH WHOM TO COLLABORATE
Present your offer in the most pleasing way to your prospective partners. Not all with accept your offer, sometimes you may have to wait till you get the right fit and keep prospecting.

STEP-5: START YOUR JOURNEY
Once your partner agrees, start your journey. Give sufficient breathing time for the business to kick start as expected, make the journey smooth. Have enough faith and confidence in your partner.

STEP-6: PERIODIC PERFORMANCE CHECK
Conduct periodic meetings with your partner/s to check the progress and evaluate if you are closely moving in the direction of meeting your objective for the collaboration. If yes, then move forward. If not, then make your partner understand

STEP-7: SCALE YOUR COLLABORATION
With the experience on where your collaboration can go right or wrong, you can now decide what kind of terms and partners suit you well. Once you have cracked it, scale it up.

STRATEGY 12

"LOCAL HERO IS THE ONE WHO IS CLOSE TO HEART"

LOCAL MARKETING

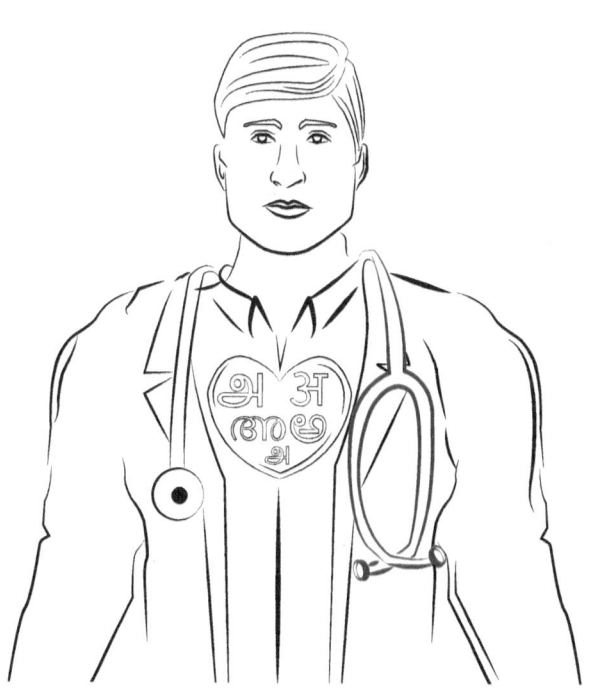

Local Hero is the Real Hero

With healthcare brands aspiring to become better day by day, their capabilities should find their own space in their own stage, instead of looking to mimic the style and strategy of other brands. With the advent of mobile technology powered by speech recognition and multilingual support, everyone in the world can access information in the language they want. Choosing regional tone and connecting with the land in native tone gives you the edge of being unique, it easily connects to your immediate audience and acts as your best resource for outreach activity because the GOOD NEWS is that there is enough content still needed in regional languages. Check if you can fill the gap and win your share of the audience.

There is a strongly visible divide among people as ruralites and urbanites. The way brands today define "reach" is different from how it is traditionally defined. It is not about from which section your audiences are all that matters is if they will consider you more close and connect well with you because of the language that you are using. Not just the language or the tonality, creating communication which is relevant to the immediate surrounding with use of local phrases will bind your brand better with your audience and that forms the crux of Local Marketing.

Regional language can become the unbreakable umbilical cord between you and your people as they get to hear what they really need to hear in their own language. This makes them connect to you instantly and you naturally get close to their heart with relatively minimum efforts.

The advent of the regional language version of international channels has once again proved that people have greater bonding with content that is given in regional language. So, if you have just English content with the motive to reach a wider set of people then maybe that only is not going to help you. English + Regional Language is the new mantra for success - you will find tonnes of examples of how people consume content when you observe web series download trends in regional language.

Also, it is an undeniable fact that every minute we are overwhelmed by content in social media, something that talks about the immediate surrounding catches our attention immediately. Similar is the case with healthcare, people in a particular geographical location may have some diseases that are common and may want to find a solution very relevant to them and that is where it becomes necessary to become a LOCAL HEALTH HERO.

6 Important aspects of Local Marketing

1 Talk to them in their language to reach their hearts

"If you talk to a man in the language he understands, that goes to his head. If you talk to him in his language that goes to his heart."
                                                            -Nelson Mandela

By talking to people in their language you build deeper bonds of trust immediately. Talking to them in the regional language doesn't stop with applying the language but also talking in the context of that particular region is even more powerful because everything changes even within regions. And, authenticity counts big.

When there is an epidemic, health-related rumors and certain other things that are specific or prevalent to your region, are things that need your attention which calls for content creation. Connect these region-specific issues and make regional content more reachable. When you offer your expertise pertaining to the regional issues that's when the consumption rate of your content will increase.

2 Know who needs you the most to become the go-to doctor

Analyze your requirements by tracking previous records, ongoing trends or small scale market research for arriving at strategies that strike the right chord in the right people. Become that one sought after medical professional who is their source of health advice and inquiry. Talk about things relating to the area of your specialization that people are looking forward to listening. Sometimes when it comes to health even those who understand English would like to confirm the message in their regional tongue before accepting and implementing it. Only with English content, you can't powerfully become the go-to doctor and a fine mix of both is required. So, count on the most prevalent issues in the region that you have zeroed to, relating to your specialty so that people can count on you for the reliable and understandable dose of information.

3   Don't let them feel alienated, set the two-way tone right!

An important characteristic of being a local health hero is also being accessible. Don't become too far-fetched that your potential patients perceive you as non-accessible. By practicing regional tone in your local marketing you are sure to attract the attention of many in your defined region and they would love to converse with you. So, create two-way communication through online and offline channels so that they can get the satisfaction of having spoken to you and clarified their doubts. Make extensive use of Local Cable TV Talk Shows, Awareness Health Gatherings, Short Talks with Q&As during camps, Webinars, Local Forums, etc. in your local marketing. Interaction & engagement creates strong and continuous bonding.

4   Play the Glocal doctor to touch more lives

The world has become a global village but there is no feeling that can beat we-feeling resulted from emotional attachment to any ethic component. If you are strong in your region and have presence with a great trust built on, then people from any part of the world belonging to that regional nativity will seek your help at the right time. Keep your local community informed about your professional accomplishments like academic achievements, research findings or case studies which will give them immense satisfaction by seeing their savior scaling heights which ultimately is going to be beneficial to the region.

5. Don't get overwhelmed by vastness, intimacy is the key to bond near or far

Community or population in any region becomes bigger as the days go by but that doesn't make the process of reaching more prospects any difficult for you. Don't get overwhelmed by the vastness. If your immediate surrounding is happy with your services, then word-of-mouth will start playing a great role, when channeled well it can show consistent results. There is enough for you, for only if you reach them the right way. Even if your reach is international, the regional momentum can give you much more leverage in unleashing your practice's fullest potential.

6. Spread awareness in the way it reaches

With proper usage, locally successful campaigning methods and mediums reach more people, more effectively. Every local medium has its own strength and may not be as effective in any other region for eg. Auto rickshaw announcements in certain rural areas are still very powerful. Awareness communication in local mediums always has the best reach as people are already tuned to those regional mediums for any major announcements, there is no chance of missing it. Local medium in the local style and regional language is the key to success.

Regional Connect is the ultimate power of any hospital brand. Among the one who has just expertise and the one who has expertise with a common ethnic attachment, it is always the latter who has a very apparent advantage in the priority list of people. Compared to other players, people who have a regional follower base will always earn the best of respect and love directly from people. The touch of real-time connection will be more fairly visible and they are the immediate audience you can win easily - even if you dream to become a renowned specialist in the world, this local audience is going to be your real brand ambassador and can make that happen. The biggest healthcare infrastructure of big brands is made use of only after a reassuring opinion given by the one who is more connected to people. The one who has the most regional connect becomes the gateway of guiding patients to the right healthcare brand at the right time even if he/she himself/herself falls short on infrastructural capability. A local player can always collaborate with other local players for the betterment of the region and also can collaborate with bigger setups for advanced care when needed by his/her people.

The emotional climate of the whole world is to stay rooted to their native culture and stage grounded to their regional self. "I am one among you" feeling is very a strong feeling and the secret to Local Marketing.

12
LOCAL MARKETING
ACTION PLAN

GOOGLE MY BUSINESS

Google My Business has become very smart & powerful. It has all the essentials necessary which can create a favourable impression about your hospital brand before a prospective patient.

6 Main things to capitalise with Google My Business

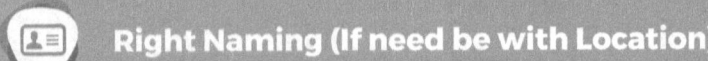
Right Naming (If need be with Location)

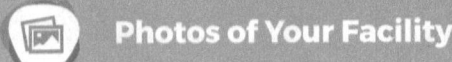
Photos of Your Facility

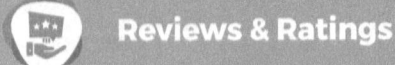
Reviews & Ratings

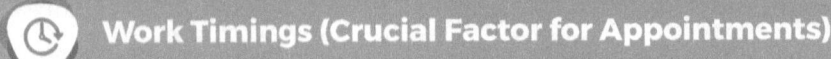
Precisely Direct to your centre with Google Maps

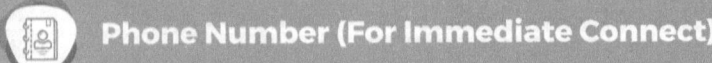
Work Timings (Crucial Factor for Appointments)

Phone Number (For Immediate Connect)

Tips : There are a lot of interesting features to explore in Google My Business like posting updates that you can explore. If you don't have a website so far then you can create a free website through Google My Business but it will have limited features only (its good for a start).

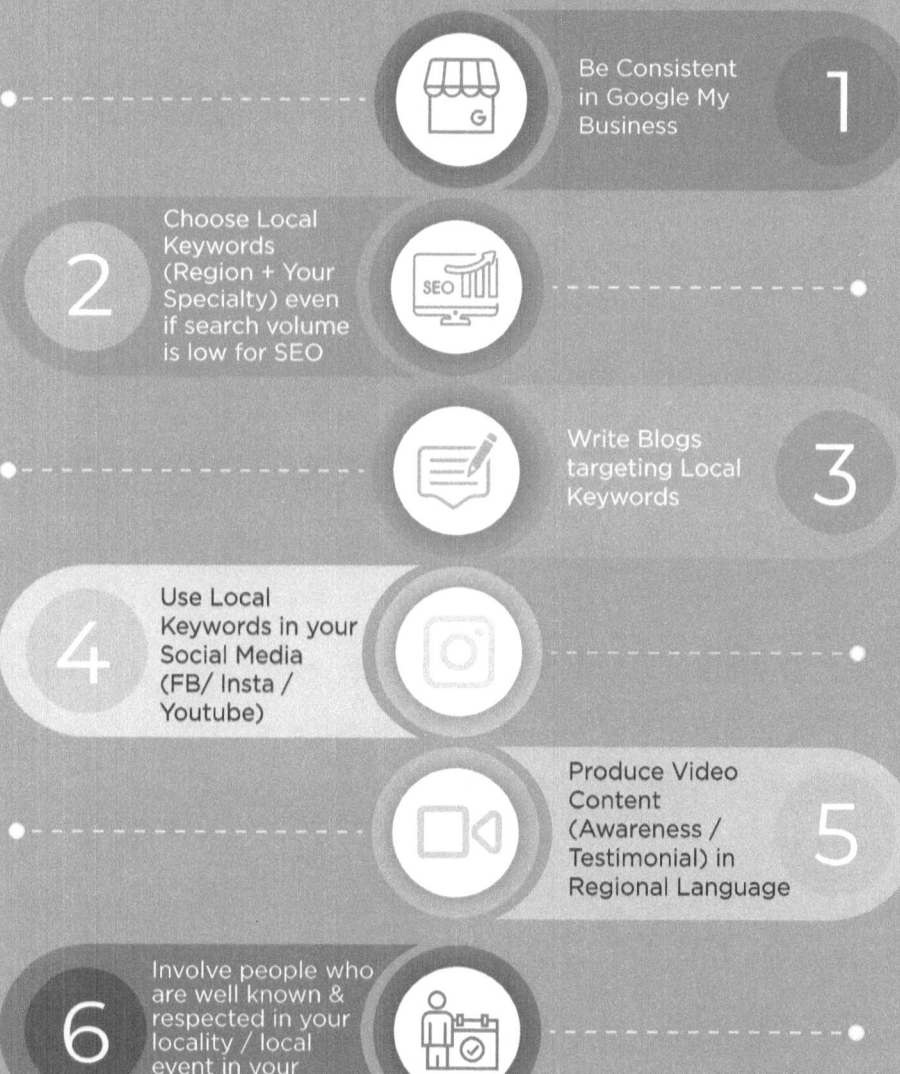

CHECKLIST FOR LOCAL MARKETING

		Yes	No
1	Do you have a clear cut Local Marketing Plan for action ?	☐	☐
2	Do you have a 12 months Local Marketing Plan?	☐	☐
3	Are people recognising your presence?	☐	☐
4	Do you get a pulse of what they are looking forward to?	☐	☐
5	Are people coming to you after they see you as a cause leader?	☐	☐
6	Are people recognising you with your specialty?	☐	☐
7	Is cause + specialty popularisation happening through your activities ?	☐	☐

CHECKLIST FOR LOCAL MARKETING

		Yes	No
8	Are you getting invites to attend local events and share your cause ?	☐	☐
9	Are you effectively leveraging your local connect mediums for promoting the cause?	☐	☐
10	Are you creating content consistently?	☐	☐
11	Is your content 80% helpful and 20% promotion in nature?	☐	☐
12	Are you leveraging your Local FREE PR support?	☐	☐
13	Are you publishing post activity report in your communication channels (Online & Offline)?	☐	☐
14	Are you documenting your Local Support Activities ?	☐	☐

6 STEP BY STEP PROCESS TO BECOME A LOCAL HERO

1. CAUSE
Select a cause dear to your Region that aligns with your specialty
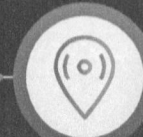

2. CHANNELS
Create Communication Channels to Reach your Region (Local TV / Local Paper / Local Outdoor Media / Direct Meet ups / FB / Youtube)
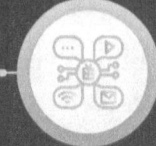

3. CONTENT
Create Content to fill these communication channels Consistently (Once a Week or Twice a week is a good frequency and later you can reduce this to once a month)

4. CONNECT
Be Accessible & connected (Direct Meet / Phone Call / Watsapp / Chat)
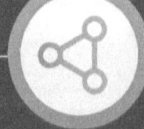

5. CONTINUE
Create Action Plan for Local Community Welfare for an year. Do good with utmost sincerity and make it known (Leverage Local PR)

6. COLLABORATE
Participate in other Local Events & promote the cause

STRATEGY 13

"YOUR NICHE IS YOUR WAY TO YOUR GLORY AND SUCCESS"

Specialty SPECIFIC

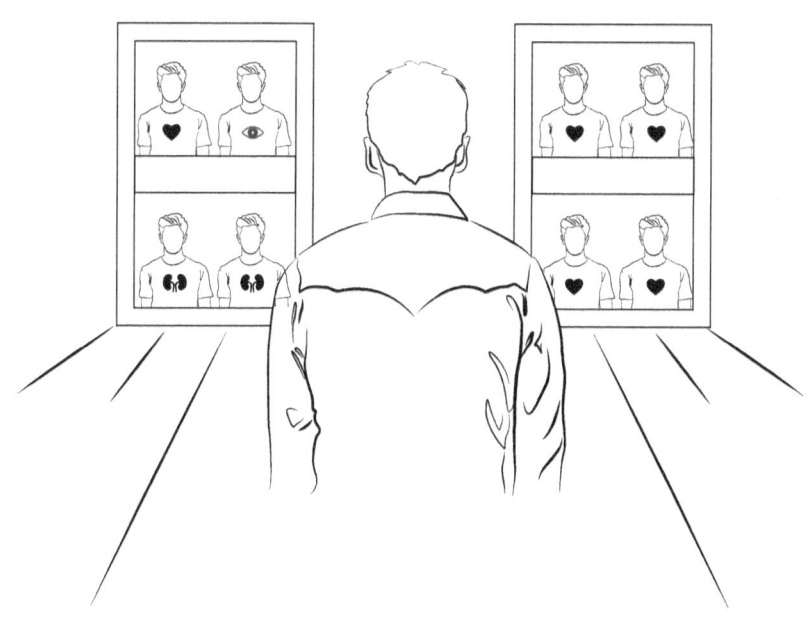

Your Strength is your Specialty

A focused, specific strength is always greater than the cumulative strength of distributed focuses from many. Specialty Specific healthcare brands always have an edge over the others because the clarity that these healthcare brands have over the others is far more possible than the rest multi-specialty hospitals. People are preferring to consult with specialists more than generalists. Today is the age of specialization and specialists in micro fields have a much bigger market today as they have a bigger scope to cater to the population in the world who needs their service. If you have a specialty-specific strength that is much more valuable today, with that you can serve more people and grow your brand globally.

People in search of specialists, travel to any part of the world to get treated. As the health complexities are increasing day by day, only a specialist keeps track of the latest happenings in the specialized field of medicine and also regularly contributes to the fraternity knowledge in various online forums and CMEs by presenting miraculous case studies. Your niche is your way to your real glory and your success. Your niche will guide you to greater heights and make you easily visible with your good work very fast. The more you travel up the pyramid, the more you will find lesser people in that area of specialization and more scope for your growth & contribution to the world.

8 Important Points to Consider in Specialty Specific Approach

1 **The right approach takes you to the right people at the right time**

Your niche is your specialized area of operation within the highly crowded market. A specialist is not meant to do generalist work. At the same time, the specialist needs to communicate the area of specialization to attract the right audience who need specialized services only. When your branding and positioning is strong and clear, you will find that you attract the right target audience that you are willing to cater to.

2 **Strategize your priorities by prioritizing your specialty in your strategies**

Make your specialty the main focus of your strategies. Market your hospital by highlighting your main specialty in every activity focused on marketing. Make your prospects reach you for the one procedure that's rarely done, which you are capable of doing. A clear cut strategy revolving specialty development should be the main focus.

3. Become the face of the specialty

Your specialty or super specialty can be known by your name, provided you establish yourself/your hospital or your personal brand as synonymous as possible to your specialty. Be the first one to educate your patient community, interact and clear the air about any taboo or misconceptions regarding the health issues pertaining to your specialty.

4. Specialty specific approach converts a red ocean to blue

As a specialty-specific hospital / personal brand the way you approach your target market will automatically take a paradigm shift. Instead of aiming big with a multi-specialty approach, aim at one and go big. If your focus is undiluted you are sure to win world attention and scale much faster than you can imagine.

5. Education relating to the specialty

Create education communication relating to your specialty. People may not be aware of the latest medical advances which can cure some of the most dangerous diseases. Preventive education will help to be aware of the deadly diseases and how to prevent them, and patient education will help the existing patients learn how to come out of the deadly clutches of the disease - using a fine combination of these in your online and offline campaigns will establish you to be the go-to source for information pertaining to your specialty. Use youtube extensively, videos reach faster in regional languages. Build a community that is highly informed.

6. Case Study relating to Specialty

Being a specialist you would have come across rare cases that are generally considered as untreatable and you would cure it through your specialized knowledge in the specialty. Such cases become important case studies that require documentation and the same has to be presented to your fraternity who learn more about it and spread light, and also those who have lost hope can find a ray of hope and come to you for getting treated. The story form of narrating case studies is very powerful when you have to reach the general public. Yes, you have to obtain permission from the patient before publishing patient experiences/testimonies.

7. Cause Leader in the Specialty

Being a specialist you have the responsibility of being a cause leader. Pick up a cause which is dear to your specialty and for which there is an actual need to help. Conduct on-ground activities and door-to-door campaigns by leveraging the strength of NGOs, govt bodies, volunteers and your own staff. Create mission numbers and achieve the numbers during the campaign. Be an exemplary cause leader that people will look up to and take inspiration from.

8. Collaborate with fraternity

Collaborate with your fraternity, success comes only when you are working together and not by working in isolation. Collaboration is necessary to share various opportunities for growth and knowledge sharing. Specialists in the same area still need major collaborations as the field of study within any specialization is very vast, specialist become super-specialists within the specialty - so a major collaboration is required always so that at the time of need to save a patient, it is definitely going to count.

We are seeing increasing trends of specialty chains evolving today which is very commonly found in areas like fertility, ophthalmology, dental, cosmetology ..etc. These specialty-specific brands are very focussed and scale well in a very short time. Specialists from India have

Specialty Specific

established brands in many countries of the world and are regularly treating patients in large numbers and it is no wonder looking at these scales of patients coming to India, flight frequency has also increased for certain geographies looking at these booming numbers to support Medical Tourism in a large way. These specialty centers are also tie-ing up with multi-specialty hospitals and take care of only that specialty, for which the infra is provided by multi-specialty. We are going to see many interesting models in this space. It will be no surprise, multi-specialty hospitals will become a multi-brand specialty center like how in a mall we get to shop from various brands under one roof, soon we will see the strong network of specialty centers coming to multi-specialty hospitals and taking care of those respective departments.

Note

13
SPECIALTY SPECIFIC
MARKETING

STEPS INVOLVED IN
SPECIALTY SPECIFIC MARKETING

STEP 01

MAIN FOCUS
Be clear about what in your specialty will be your main focus as each specialty is an ocean on its own.

STEP 02

CREATE SPECIALTY COMMUNICATION
Create helpful awareness communication collaterals like brochures / leaflets / posters / videos /blogs / local TV programs, etc. Answer Q&As online on various topics revolving around your main areas of focus.

STEP 03

MAKE YOUR BRAND SYNONYMOUS WITH YOUR SPECIALTY
When people look for information on that specific area of your specialty your information should be the first point of contact that helps the munderstand the subject better.
You should be their first teacher.

STEP 04

PAIR UP WITH A CAUSE
Align with a cause which is dear to your specialty and create camps and awareness programs collaborating with other NGOs / social organisations

STEP 05
SHARE YOUR CASE STUDY
A specialist is a subject matter expert and people from the fraternity will want to learn from your expertise, share case studies in CMEs. Also give hope to patients with case studies in story form.

STEP 06
DO REAL GOOD
Conduct camps / counselling sessions which should really help people and should not become a marketing gimmick to promote your hospital. If people understand we really care about them, then we should know there is scarcity for sincerity and we will be rewarded duly with trust.

STEP 07
EXPAND YOUR AUDIENCE
Keep yourself engaged with activities pertaining to specialty specific awareness programs. Partner with players who can introduce you to their audience.

STEP 08
SCALE YOUR GROWTH
There is a great demand for specialists. Collaborate as an individual brand or as an organisational brand with other hospitals and centres where there is a need for your specialty specific expertise. Chart out a mutual growth plan and scale great heights.

Note

STRATEGY 14

"CREATE YOUR OWN TRIBE AND LEAD THEM"

BUILD YOUR AUDIENCE

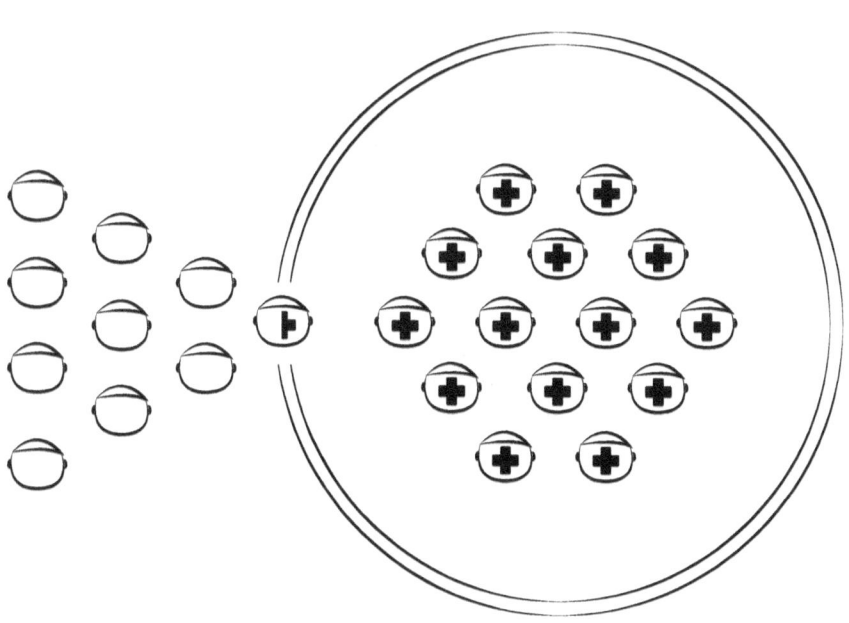

Build your tribe and Lead them

Brands that are starting to come to the light or those that have reworked their strategies always feel anxious about where they are going to pool their audience from. Creating one's own bunch of audience, most importantly creating them organically can be one daunting task for most of the nascent beings into the branding world. Having a follower base who is looking forward to engaging with the brand is important than just having a random flowing crowd stop by you.

Take any healthcare brand that you think is iconic, look into its journey of having created its own audience base. A few cult brands always have their audience base to their advantage. Also, a well-defined action plan followed by the strategy for identifying, attracting and preserving your own audience base is important. This can only tell you where your audience stream is coming from, so you cater better to them and keep satisfaction levels high.

People are silently begging to be led. They expect the utmost solidarity from their leader, they expect to receive the answers from the brands close to them even for which others might have answered, still, the answer from their trusted brands ensures confidence.

Building your brand audience requires a lot of patience and dedication. The initial journey will be very difficult as there will be replies from people who may not like you and may put you down. That's where consistency plays. Be consistent in your communication through various online and offline mediums, create useful content that people need at that time.

Talk about taking precautions during rainy season as the rainy season approaches or taking precautions against a pandemic or changing your lifestyle when you have already undergone heart bypass surgery etc. You can talk about varied things, but make sure if you stick to one branch of specialty, your reach will be much faster. Your specialty will also define your audience. When there is consistent content from you via videos, blogs, local meetups, etc people will start interacting with you and start thanking you for some valuable information that might have saved their life or the lives of their dear ones. And thus, you start developing your strong brand patrons who will multiply over a period of time. You will be a strong influencer in the lives of those you touch through your content and you may not even know who all are they.

Points to Note

1 **The treasure you seek is seeking you now. Are you ready?**

Gone are the times where you knocking your prospect's door is the only way to reach them. Now it is the time to be the authoritative brand and rule the market. It is a less utilized secret that if the world knows how worth-it you are, it will come running to you for information, service, and everything that's to do with you relating to healthcare. The first step to claiming your own audience set is to create value without expecting any returns. As people start realizing the value you are providing, they will want to test your intentions, but, be firm. Your utmost sincerity in public health can only make you a true leader leading a tribe.

2 **Utilize your invitation to cut across the crowd**

Being in places where your audience is present, delivering a message that they want to hear the most, is the only way to cut across the crowd through consistent efforts that last a lifetime and more to make your healthcare brand more rooted in the market. This happens naturally when you have carved your way to cut through the clutter and make sense to the world out there.

When you do so, the people whom you think your brand might need, will now need your brand. Building an audience will help you serve those who really deserve it. Your brand audience will create the support you require and bring in clarity towards achieving your roadmaps.

3 **Analyze anticipations and deliver**

Analyze anticipations that your prospects have in general or specific to your own loyal base. Tracking what they are asking for is important to deliver to perfection. Brands today are cracking the pulse of the audience every moment; each nuanced move of your audience base can have a role for your brand to play in. A simple step of doing so is to study the search patterns that you may come across. Cater to the best possible needs and be there to engage your audience in demanding times. By anticipating and delivering what they require from time to time you stay relevant to them.

4. Follow a clear road-map

Understand who is your target audience and also analyze who exactly became your audience. If this can be deciphered, you will know who is likely to become your audience in the near future, with this wonderful insight you can build your tribe stronger and better.

See wherever they have their most presence in, for eg: for dermatologists who treat mostly teenagers to early adults , instagram might be the best platform to catch their quality audience. Of course, it can always grow or segue to other platforms or stream from one. Look where you can intersect your service and knowledge base to their engagement pattern. Since we are exposed to an overwhelming amount of information thrown at us, we need to make a way into what people really want to consume. By becoming desirable you become compelling and then people associate with your brand even smoothly.

5. An influencer can create massive impact

By attracting an audience you become their influencer, which means your audience will listen to you dedicatedly and will do what you say. your words will have a profound effect on their life and they will make necessary changes in their lifestyle if they truly follow you. When you become an influencer you have a major responsibility in advising what is right and beneficial to people as your words will be directly taken into action by your audience. Influence them to do the right things to live a healthy life which will only add up to your brand audience vouching for you of their success.

6. Start with One Medium and then become omnipresent

When you are starting to build your audience, start with one medium. Over a period, through consistency and quality work you will develop an audience for you and then start leveraging other platforms to disseminate your brand content and your brand audience who are already present in those mediums will do the work of propagating your communication to the like-minded people who are likely to become your audience.

Sacrifice and sincerity are the building blocks of the audience who will do anything for you. And at the same time, you have a major responsibility to lead your audience, they trust you and you should never misuse their trust. Building your reputation to building an audience takes a lot of time and to break it, it takes a moment. Always do good for your tribe.

Note

14
BUILD YOUR AUDIENCE

7 STEP PROCESS TO
BUILD & GROW YOUR AUDIENCE

01 MAKE YOUR MISSION THEIR MISSION
Declare your mission in life and how it is relevant to help those who are suffering from that particular disease / complication and why tit is necessary to spread this message. And more importantly why they should support to make a difference in someone's life

02 ENGAGE WITH PROOF
Share more information in various formats, videos in regional languages are the most easy to reach a vast majority of people. Keep your content relevant to the topic and your audience. Give timely proof of how your content is helping people live better with social proof (testimonies)

03 BE TRUSTWORTHY
You cant act to be sincere, you have to be sincere. Nothing builds trust more than sincerity. Make it very clear. Helping people with right content should be your primary objective. Your promotion will happen automatically. As you build trust people are smart enough to know how to get the most from you by availing your services.

04 GIVE SIMPLE STEPS TO FOLLOW
Create content which people can easily put into action. You now know why Tik Tok is so famous. Your education content has to be simple and easily implementable (for eg. simple diet tips / exercises).

7 STEP PROCESS TO
BUILD & GROW YOUR AUDIENCE

05 REMIND THEM OF THEIR ENEMY
Remind your audience time and again with proof about the health enemies and how to safeguard your health from them

06 REMIND THEM THE REWARD
Show proofs of how people following the instructions and advise / preventive measures are leading a happy life

07 MAKE EXIT DIFFICULT
You should be so good and informative. They should find it difficult to leave you. You have to become their integral content which they consume when it comes to those topics that you discuss.

Note

STRATEGY 15

"KNOW YOURSELF BEFORE OTHERS KNOW YOU"

REPUTATION MANAGEMENT

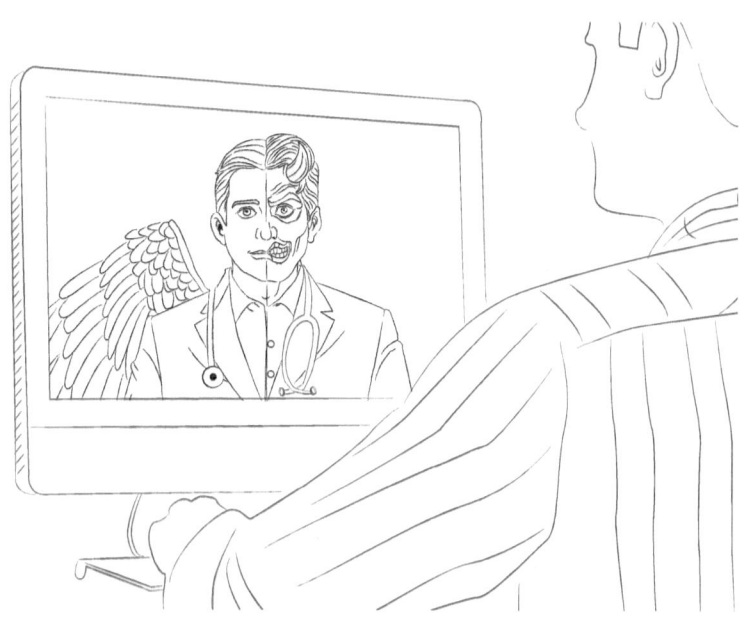

Your Reputation Precedes You

It is the era of smart patients, who are well informed, who have a perspective of their own and want to tell the world that they too have an opinion.

Doctors and healthcare brands today are thrown vulnerable to opinions every second and minute. But the ability to convert it into power or weakness, lies with the brand itself. There are techniques to craft your image in your environment. A lot of it is a natural way of response not only in a way that defends your core values but becomes a flag bearer of it. Like we discussed, these patient discussions about your brand are in online or offline needs to be well engaged with. Managing reputation is one of the greatest responsibilities of any healthcare brand today. When reputation is sealed right, then the stakeholder management strategies from all ends become very easy. All that the hospital brands have to realize is that each act impacts! And so, if right attention is paid to the value you are creating to your patients, your reputation goes self-managed and the good you create heals the world.

8 Important aspects to consider in Reputation Management

1. They are all talking about you, are you listening?

Your patients and all your fraternity members have their own voice, their own opinion. Now, with multiple channels, there are enough opportunities for one to express. So, listen to them clearly and decide to reply or fill gaps in your operations. Today a brand that listens to its patients and responds proactively without exhibiting ignorance or indifference is way more desirable than just any other brand.

2. The word of that your brand has is a reverberation of your reputation

In order to manage your reputation well, you have to first understand how much an un-maintained reputation is costing. Today nobody opts for a healthcare brand over another because it is near their home, there is a process that every patient undergoes before even entering the premise of your practice. And that process involves only your reputation and discussions around it. The number of new patients you are acquiring, the new workforce you are attracting are all a result of your reputation.

3 Don't let the not so good decide your brand image

Maintain that balance for better digital health of your healthcare brand. People who have had good experiences with your brand consider it to be normal, so they fail to express it, so, make good opinions also reach people. There are enough amount of good experiences that your brand kindles, but are they evoking a ripple effect? Or are they being left alone in vacuum unaffecting your brand image positively. This decides the overall mood of all reviews and word-of-mouth your brand has been off-late generating. Maintaining the equilibrium irrespective of the nature of flowing feedbacks is necessary for a healthcare brand.

4 Don't take your reputation for granted!

Saying, people will keep expressing what they feel and you cannot control, is just an excuse you are giving to your brand value. If you have a justification tell the world, defend your brand or even express a moment of gratitude when there is an opinion out there. Even if a healthcare brand unintentionally leaves its reputation unmonitored, it can cost the management more than what anybody can actually think. After all, today everything is accessible and measurable at the touch of a button. So, every decision now is taken based on somebody else's decision. This is exactly why you can't leave your reputation to a mere philosophical attitude. Take charge now!

5 Understand that reviews are a package and baggage. Address the good and the bad!

Every healthcare brand faces its own share of good and otherwise, it is only wise to face the "otherwise" too. Managing your reputation is not a tedious task if you get to know how vital it is to your brand image and reputation.

Take all the contemporary brands in any industry who are doing constantly well with super engagement rates from its target audience. You are certain to notice one thing in common- they speak to them, not just respond. Now, engagement and most importantly meaningful engagement is the key to getting ahead with review management.

6. Derive feedbacks from opinions

You should rather thank the mechanism of online reviews to rework your service value proposition. There is definitely an issue with your overall service that's taking your business downhill or is plateauing your patient count. It might be a tedious process for you to find out the gaps that your business is leaving, but the online medium thankfully opens up the Pandora's Box for you to find the treasure. Hear what people say and use it to your advantage to deliver better care.

7. No substitute to Transparency and Genuineness

It is no art of elites or rocket science to take action and manage your reputation. It is a simple act like a real-time conversation with your patients and colleagues. Be as transparent as possible. People never want their brands to be 100% perfect because they know ideally, it can never be. But everybody wants a healthcare brand that truly cares. They prefer the one that strives hard for the patient's well-being amidst all odd, so be transparent and involve your true brand loyalists when there is any good they can do. Your core values are the spine for your reputation.

8. Make sure each feel-good story created in your hospital heals the world

A lot of your reputation goes fine and self-managed by making the good reach far and beyond. The world loves to indulge in true goodness and magic that a healthcare organization creates.

Reputation Management

Being a healthcare brand of today's day and age concentrates more on occupying the positive headspace of your target audience.

There is no excuse for not managing your reputation online. I remember one instance where a brand got a negative comment in a popular online forum and even before the brand could reply there were half a dozen comments defending the brand - Do you know who posted those comments? Yes, online word-of-mouth agents, patients who experienced the "moments of truth," who could not agree with that negative comment. They all started sharing their side of the story with the brand and said how the individual who wrote the bad comment may be misguided or wrongly informed about the brand. Your tribe will defend you, build you, and make you reach your goal.

Note

15

REPUTATION MANAGEMENT
ACTION PLAN

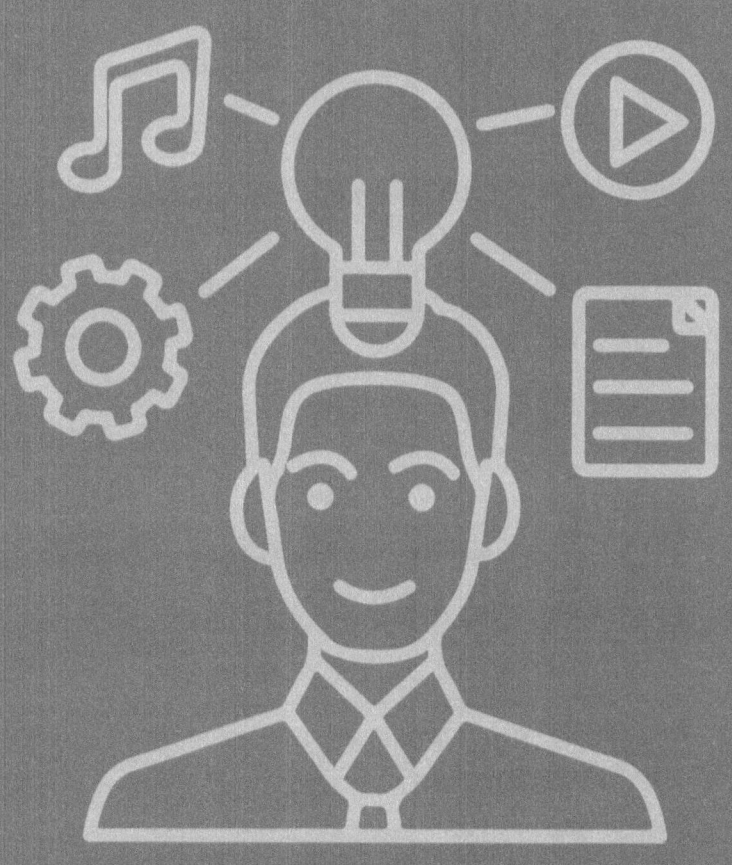

ONLINE REPUTATION MANAGEMENT (ORM) CHECKLIST

Yes No

1 What are your goals for ORM ?

- Just reducing negative reviews ☐ ☐
- Increasing positive impressions ☐ ☐
- Engaging with patients online ☐ ☐

2 What are the platforms you are concentrating on?

- Google Reviews ☐ ☐
- Your Website ☐ ☐
- Online Review Sites ☐ ☐
- Directory Sites ☐ ☐

3 Do you read your reviews daily and respond? ☐ ☐

4 Do you have a team set to monitor Online Reputation? ☐ ☐

5 Do your doctors also participate in clarifying specific issues? ☐ ☐

ONLINE REPUTATION MANAGEMENT (ORM) CHECKLIST

		Yes	No
6	Do you observe trends in your complaints and rectify?	☐	☐
7	Do you learn from your reviews and improvise your operations?	☐	☐
8	Do you encourage patients to share reviews?	☐	☐
9	How often does your team reply diligently to reviews?	☐	☐
10	Do you have a feedback book in your hospital lobby?	☐	☐
11	Do you have a wall of "Thank you doctor" notes?	☐	☐

STEP BY STEP INSTRUCTIONS TO TAKE CONTROL OF YOUR HOSPITAL REPUTATION ONLINE

1. REGISTER IN GOOGLE MY BUSINESS

Get your business registered in Google My Business with clear direction and contact information mentioned. If you are not creating it, to your surprise someoneelse would have created it - so claim your name and address. Unless you have control you cannot monitor and reply effectively. Not being there is not an excuse.

2. ENCOURAGE PATIENTS TO REVIEW

Patients who are happy about your service and thank you for the same, you can direct them if they wish to review in Google My Business. Why GMB? Because that is the most trusted review spot now which people trust. Note: There should be no forceful reviews obtained.

3. USE THE POSITIVE

For positive reviews thank them and publish them in your hospital waiting area, website & social media. Thank positive reviews addressing their name. Publish the positive reviews only with the permission of patients.

4. REPLY THE NEGATIVE

For negative reviews, reply to them appropriately depending on whether the mistake is on their side or your side or is it a fake review just to spoil your reputation.

5. GET GOOGLE ALERTS

Get your brand name registered in Google Alerts to get an instant update whenever there is any information about your brand on Google. Whenever your brand is mentioned anywhere in the internet where google has access, you will get mail notification instantly - this will save any big damage.

STEP BY STEP INSTRUCTIONS TO TAKE CONTROL OF YOUR HOSPITAL REPUTATION ONLINE

6

NICE REPLY FORMATS

Have a standard tone of replies, it should not look mechanical but polite and graceful. The tone should be highly encouraging the brand patrons. As the scenario demands you can break the monotony and improvise on these messages periodically. The idea is it should not look like it is a machine reply but a human replying.

7

NO FAKE POSITIVE

Don't encourage fake positive reviews. Don't think that you can fool google, the algorithm is becoming more smarter everyday and also you cannot fool people-they can make out between a fake one and a genuine one.

8

ACT WHAT YOU LEARN

Follow strict discipline while understanding the reviews-both negative and positive. People will love a brand if they see their suggestions are taken in a right way instead of being stubborn. Bridge the gaps which are highlighted in your negative reviews.

9

BE PREPARED FOR A BAD DAY

Even if you have organically gathered positive reviews, you cannot remain silent. You have to be prepared for a bad day which can be a willful act of someone. When you have enough positive and very minimal negative you will score high overall and that counts a lot.

Psychology of Review Reading Audience

STEP 01 — **OVERALL RATING MATTERS**
People always consider overall rating to be the main factor to get favourable impression to opt a brand

STEP 02 — **NEGATIVE CAN BE SUBJECTIVE**
People understand not all brands will be free from negative reviews, which can arise due to subjective experience even with a good brand

STEP 03 — **IS NEGATIVE TRUE**
People will judge the truthfulness of the negative review with the replies that you give to respond

STEP 04 — **FASTER REPLY**
People like brands that reply fast. But you can take time to carefully analyse and reply in certain critical situations.

STEP 05 — **POSITIVE REVIEWS ANALYSIS**
They will also want to know if you are thanking those who have given positive reviews and what exactly are the positive reviews about. Does it look like fake? Or they seem to be genuine.

Psychology of Review Reading Audience

STEP 06

NEGATIVE ABOUT WHAT COUNTS

People would try to understand what these negative reviews are revolving around - if its about staff / behaviour / hygiene / infra - then it's not so serious and may be subjective. If it is about a death due to negligence, money mindedness, wrong prescription, etc then it is a very dangerous thing.

STEP 07

POSITIVE ABOUT WHAT COUNTS

Also people would like to understand what these positive reviews are all about. If the positive reviews complement staff / behaviour / hygiene / infra - then it can create a neutral effect as some of these are subjective experiences even if they find negative on these areas. If the reviews complement the doctor, their style of practice, the timely support that saved them from pain and agony - then this will carry more weight in forming a favourable impression about your brand.

STEP 08

MEET PRIMARY PURPOSE

If the primary purpose of approaching a hospital is to find a healthcare partner that have been trusted for their core values is found then the job is done

BEST WAYS TO TACKLE NEGATIVE REVIEWS

 **ADDRESS THEM AT THE EARLIEST**

- *Address them with their name*

 **IF IT IS YOUR MISTAKE / SOMETHING UNCLEAR**

- *Start by asking for their contact details if you don't have / if you have contact details call them & understand*
- *Accept to correct it. Take it offline immediately.*
- *After the issue is solved you can ask them to give a positive review right below their negative review*
- *If it is something that the patient is not convinced about then you can leave this subject, with your reply as the last.*
- *If the patient again goes back online with more negative, You can best write a convincing apology note, point out areas where you would be willing to support.*

 IF IT IS A FAKE REVIEW

- *Ask for patient details & other specifics*
- *Mostly they will not respond. If they do, then ask for further details more politely*
- *You will not get a reply and you can conclude politely by saying we doubt if it was a fake review (do not conclude unless you are sure). You can also use statements like-We do not find any record of such patient in our register or can you help us with more details*

 **IF IT IS NOT YOUR MISTAKE**

- *Ask for patient details & other specifics. Verify the incident thoroughly before replying*
- *Quote your side of the incident, justify and defend gracefully.*
- *Accept to correct in areas where it may seem appropriate*
- *Stay transparent with dates, figures and facts.*
- *If people get mad, do not lose your cool. Keep defending as it may seem appropriate but not more than 3 exchanges.*

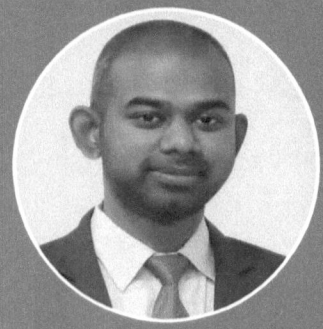

Mohammed Ilias

Healthcare Branding & Marketing Strategist
BCC Healthcare

Author, Trainer, Speaker, Market Creator & Ethical Marketer

www.mdilias.com

Mohammed Ilias is an International Healthcare Branding and Marketing Strategist successfully running BCC Healthcare - an integrated healthcare branding and marketing agency with presence in India, UAE and Srilanka. He works closely with Hospitals, Celebrity Doctors, Pharma Companies, Labs, Medical Equipment Manufacturers. With a decade of experience in healthcare industry he has served over 100+ brands to achieve better presence and deliver enriched brand communication in the market.

His mastery over the art of amalgamating strong marketing strategies and aesthetically rich creatives to bring out campaigns that hit the right chord at the right time in the right target audience is remarkable.

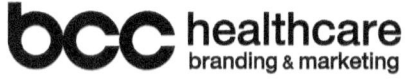

www.bcchealthcarebranding.com

BCC Healthcare is a branding and marketing agency working extensively on healthcare segment with a presence in India, Sri Lanka and UAE. We have developed a number of successful campaigns for various established hospitals and other healthcare brands.

Healthcare is our specialty too, we serve as brand partners for numerous Healthcare Brands. Our expertise in Healthcare Marketing is a result of our deep insights driven by experience and derived from market study & analysis. We understand your target audience as much as you do. We find that one USP of our client to make them cut through the noise and stand out in a market overcrowded by competitors.

What we do:

We create tailor-made campaigns for our clients, our repertoire as an agency extends from creating quick brand deliverables, digital brand assets to immensely impactful TV commercials. We add value to our clients through the following services:

- 360-degree Healthcare branding and marketing campaign
- Engaging Digital Marketing Strategies (National & International)
- Specialty Specific Content Marketing
- SEO friendly Hospital Website
- Signages as per NABH norms
- Techno-Creative Products
- Outdoor & Indoor Hospital Branding
- TV Commercial
- Educative Doctor Branding & Interview Videos
- Brand Souvenirs
- CME Management and Promotion
- Medical Tourism outreach Digital Support

www.ingramcontent.com/pod-product-compliance
Lightning Source LLC
Chambersburg PA
CBHW020859180526
45163CB00007B/2566